CHAKRAS & SELF-CARE

CHAKRAS
& SELF-CARE

ACTIVATE THE HEALING
POWER OF CHAKRAS
WITH EVERYDAY RITUALS

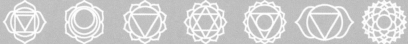

AMBI KAVANAGH

FOREWORD BY POPPY JAMIE

ZEITGEIST · NEW YORK

Published in the United States by Zeitgeist, an imprint of Zeitgeist™,
a division of Penguin Random House LLC, New York.

penguinrandomhouse.com

Zeitgeist™ is a trademark of Penguin Random House LLC

ISBN: 9780593196687
Ebook ISBN: 9780593196748

Cover art © by Ramziya Khusnullina/Shutterstock.com
Interior art © by Ju Alaris/Shutterstock.com
Author photo © Jon Hammond Hagan
Book design by Aimee Fleck

Printed in China

5 7 9 10 8 6 4

First Edition

DEDICATED TO
MY HUSBAND, KEVIN,
OUR SON, ASHER,
AND MY TEACHER NOELLE:
MY CHAKRA-BALANCING COHORTS

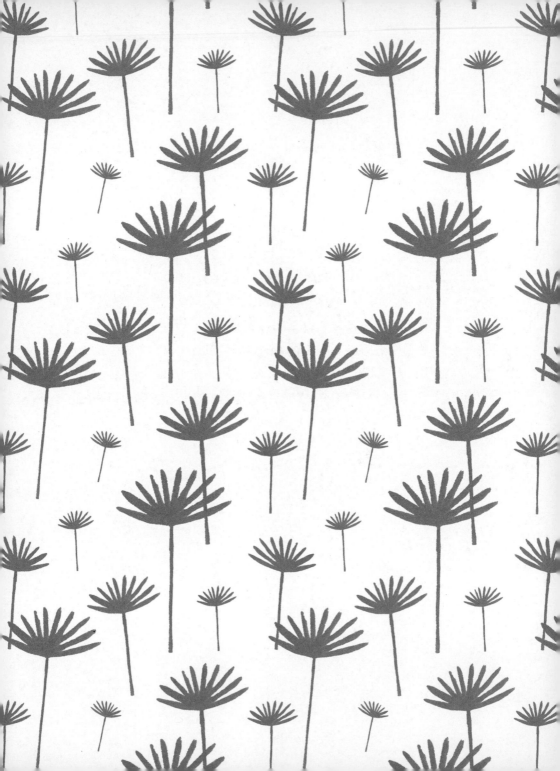

TABLE OF CONTENTS

FOREWORD

At its core, self-care is the deliberate act of valuing our own mental, emotional, spiritual, and physical health. It is rooted in self-love and having the ability to check in with ourselves and meet ourselves exactly where we are at. Unfortunately, the true meaning of self-care has gotten lost in translation. We see it portrayed everywhere as a modern trend with lavish bubble baths, overadvertised subscription boxes, and celery juice. In our nonstop information-overloaded world, we often get sucked into this and lose track of real self-care as we prioritize getting "likes" and keeping busy above our own needs. So it's not surprising that we find ourselves a bit lost and in desperate need of guidance when we try to take control of our health and happiness.

This is where *Chakras & Self-Care* comes in. Consider it your guide to building, nourishing, and balancing your well-being as you navigate modern life. Combining practical rituals with the science and philosophy from thousands of years, it teaches you about the power of balancing your energy system, or your chakras. You'll learn to connect with your inner guidance system and unlock the wisdom you carry in your body. Preventative health begins when the reconnection process starts, and your mind, body, and soul move in harmony.

This book is also a manifestation of its author, Ambi Kavanagh. A spectacular and much-needed voice in this field, Ambi spent years as a lawyer before becoming a leader in the wellness industry (even before there was such an "industry") using modalities such as sound healing, astrology, Reiki, and life coaching. Grounded in her own experiences, she has a unique ability to heal, mend, and leave you shining from within.

As you turn the pages, you might begin by opening one of your chakras under Ambi's guidance, or perhaps trying one of her rituals for releasing what no longer serves you. Over time, you'll likely find yourself incorporating more and more practices into your daily life—and that's when the rejuvenating healing truly takes off.

I am excited as you embark on your healing journey to learn about the most balanced, awake, and aligned version of yourself. You are not only in safe hands, but in magical, healing ones.

POPPY JAMIE

Founder, Happy Not Perfect

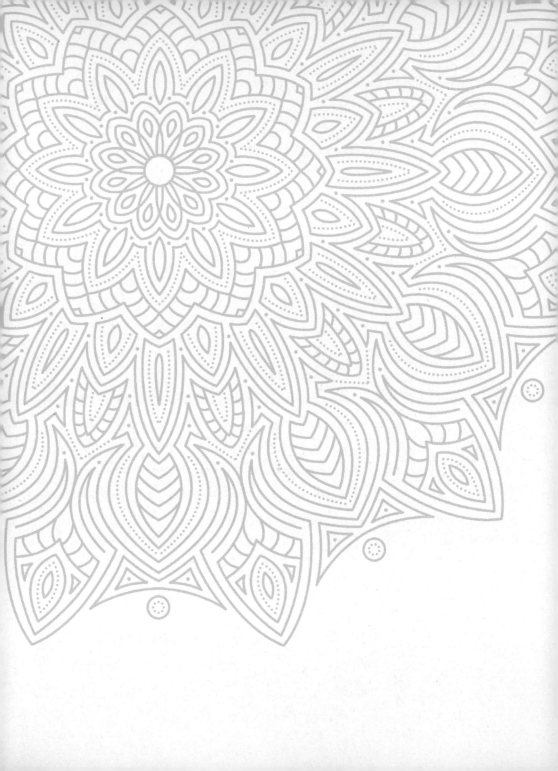

INTRODUCTION

THERE IS DEEP WISDOM WITHIN
OUR VERY FLESH, IF WE CAN ONLY
COME TO OUR SENSES AND FEEL IT.

Elizabeth A. Behnke

What if everything you needed to be your best self—mind, body, and soul—was already within you? Imagine if this wisdom contained not only remedies for your life but also preventative practices, so you would have fewer problems to deal with. How different would life be if you could harness this knowledge to experience more peace of mind, better physical health, and a sense of alignment, fulfillment, and purpose? In this book, we explore how the age-old wisdom of the chakra system can help you achieve this and more.

Chakra, which comes from ancient Sanskrit, means "spinning wheel of light." The chakra system is composed of seven main energy wheels that regulate our energetic bodies. Our ancestors intuitively understood and worked with their energetic bodies and the rhythms and seasons of nature. The good news is, this knowledge and practice are not limited to the past. And we need them more in our modern-day lives than ever before. Just like our ancestors, we also can live in alignment with the lunar cycles and Mother Nature to tap into our natural biorhythms—the body cycles that regulate our health, emotions, and intellect.

In today's hectic and often stressful world, the wheels of our energetic body are often compromised to the detriment of our physical body and, indeed, our life. And while we spend time, money, and energy taking care of our physical body, we often overlook our energetic body and underestimate the important role it plays in our overall well-being. If we want optimum health, we need to give more care to our energetic body. While modern medicine has made many advances that have changed our lives, it has also inadvertently diminished our innate ability to self-heal. Many diseases actually stem from "dis-ease," or a disconnect between the mind, body, and soul, caused by blockages in the energetic body. We all know that prevention is better than a cure, and many of our ailments are preventable by consciously working with the chakra system of self-care.

I discovered the chakra system soon after my spiritual awakening in 2008 and have since studied and worked with the chakra system of self-care to bring more order, balance, and harmony to my life. It was one of the biggest lessons and teachings I've received— and it turned my life around. (I credit this awakening and the journey that followed with helping me naturally conceive and birth my healthy baby boy in my early forties!) As a Reiki master, sound healer, astrologer, and life coach, I have shared this knowledge with hundreds of my clients in our work together. I have seen firsthand the positive impact chakra self-care has had on their lives, helping them to overcome health issues, be more energized, enjoy peace of mind, align with their true purpose, and have more self-confidence. As a result, they were able to attract the right people and make positive decisions in difficult situations. It has been incredible to witness the power of this practice.

This book will help you harness these timeless teachings so you experience more balance, healing, and harmony. In the first part of the book, we explore each of the seven main chakras and their function in your life. You'll also learn about crystals and essential oils that help open each chakra, and we will cover goddess archetypes to help you reach each chakra's highest potential. I'll also provide you with exercises and meditations, including a chakra visualization meditation to help you connect to these energy centers, and then I will lead you through a step-by-step activation meditation that will help open each chakra so its energy flows freely.

The second part of the book covers practices for both daily and seasonal chakra balancing, and includes remedies and recipes, as well as rituals, affirmations, and meditations. They will help you learn how to incorporate this timeless wisdom into your everyday life.

My sincere hope in writing this book is to help you become more connected to yourself and to the natural world. As you learn about the chakra system and the workings of your energy body, you will learn to appreciate your innate power, and it will transform your life. I encourage you to take your time with the book; soak it all up, journal about your experiences with the meditations and rituals, and revisit chapters as needed. With the deep wisdom of the chakras within you, you will be empowered to enjoy a healthier, happier, more aligned existence; embrace your true essence; enjoy your loved ones; and relish the natural world and a better quality of life.

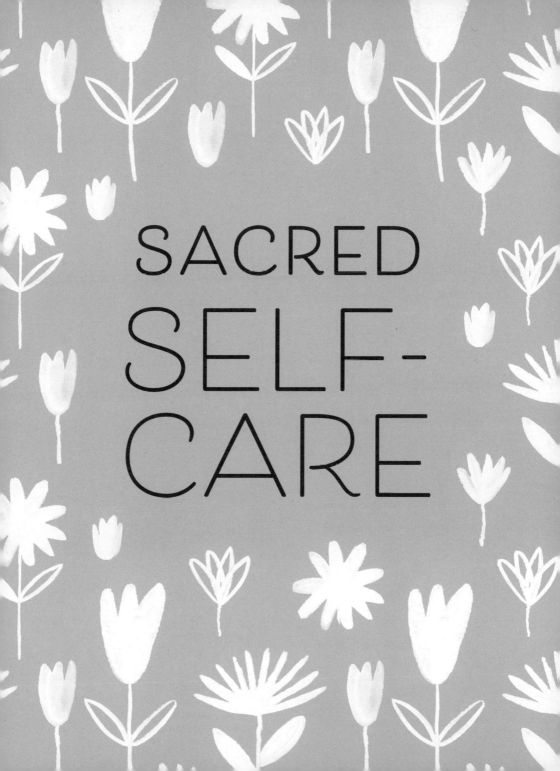

SACRED SELF-CARE

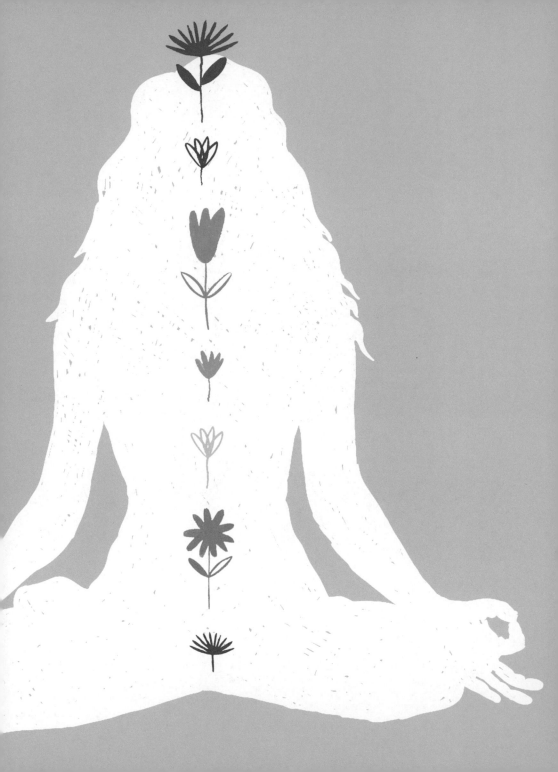

ONE

CHAKRA FOUNDATION

> **THE FLOW OF ENERGY
> THROUGH A SYSTEM ACTS
> TO ORGANIZE THAT SYSTEM.**
>
> *Harold Morowitz*

In this chapter, I will introduce you to the history of the chakras and help you build your foundation of knowledge. You will learn about the seven major chakras, the many key concepts and terms associated with chakra energy healing, and the tools that you can harness to begin your journey. There will also be a practical exercise to help you connect to and evaluate your chakras, so you can begin understanding how to restore any energetic imbalances.

WHAT IS A CHAKRA?

As mentioned in the introduction, chakra is a Sanskrit word meaning "spinning wheel." Sanskrit is the ancient Vedic language used in India, and the term chakra was first described in Vedic scriptures thousands of years ago. In ancient texts called the Vedas, the chakras were described as being connected by nadis (Sanskrit for "rivers"), which allowed prana (Sanskrit for "life force") to flow through our bodies.

Many ancient spiritual texts use metaphors and symbolism as part of their teachings. The Vedas used land as a metaphor for the physical body, with the seven main chakras as different parts of the land, and the nadis as the rivers that connected and flowed between them. In order for the land to flourish, each of the seven parts needed to be watered by the rivers that flowed freely and fully without hindrance.

Using this symbolism, the scriptures taught that in order for us to experience optimum life force, to have the best physical and emotional health, and to flourish, all the chakras needed to be open and spinning, thus allowing energy to flow freely throughout the body. If any of the chakras were not performing optimally, energetic imbalance or blockage could ensue, leading to physical, emotional, spiritual, and life issues.

While the first references to chakras were found in Hindu scriptures, the teachings of Buddhists, Tibetans, Mayans, and Kabbalists, among others, acknowledge the chakras and refer to a similar system in their teachings. As humanity has evolved, we have explored wellness outside the realms of traditional medicine and, in many cases, looked to our ancestors for age-old solutions to modern-day problems. Practices such as yoga, which also originated in India, have become popular, and slowly but surely, the teachings of the chakra system of self-care have come to the forefront as age-old tools for holistic healing.

IS CHAKRA ENERGY REAL?

Many people may be skeptical of energy healing and perhaps think of it as being "woo-woo" or quackery. Maybe you are even a little unconvinced of its merits right now. However, energy healing has become more widely practiced outside of alternative healing and has been integrated into modern medicine. For example, doctors use forms of energy healing such as vibrational sound energy or infrared lasers for treatment, and some hospitals offer Reiki, an energy healing practice. These treatments are even covered by many medical health insurance policies as alternative treatments similar to acupuncture, which provides healing using fine needles placed at specific points along the body to bring energy into alignment. As you can see, energy healing is becoming increasingly more mainstream.

Energy is a word that gets thrown around a lot in the self-help world. It is the subject of many motivational quotes and some humorous memes, so it may seem a bit of a vague and meaningless term, but this is far from the truth. In short, energy is formally defined by science as both "matter," which has the potential to cause changes, and the capacity of a physical system to do "work." Science explains that energy cannot be created or destroyed, only changed. Science also dictates that everything, including the chair you are sitting on, and indeed your body, is made of energy.

Each of our bodies is also surrounded by a field of constantly changing energy. For our bodies to be capable of "work" and for certain aspects (e.g., body parts or areas of life) to work, our energy will need to operate in a particular manner. For the purposes of engaging our chakra system, when we talk about energy, we mean the prana—life force—that flows through our bodies and allows us to function.

THE SEVEN MAJOR CHAKRAS

The chakra system is a network of channels consisting of different energy wheels. While there are over a hundred different chakras, seven of these are the main chakras that form the foundation of our energy bodies. These start from the base of the spine, and travel through to the crown of the head. Each of these seven chakras relates to specific organs within the body, as well as various emotional, psychological, and spiritual states.

As you can see on the following page, the root chakra is at the base of the spine and farther up is the sacral chakra, which is found around two inches below the belly button. Then there is the solar plexus chakra in the abdomen. At the chest is the heart chakra. Moving up, in the neck is the throat chakra. Between the eyebrows is the third eye, or brow chakra. And finally, at the top of the head, we have the suitably named crown chakra.

SAHASRARA

THE CROWN CHAKRA

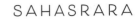

AJNA

THE BROW CHAKRA

VISHUDDHA

THE THROAT CHAKRA

ANAHATA

THE HEART CHAKRA

MANIPURA

THE SOLAR PLEXUS CHAKRA

SWADHISTHANA

THE SACRAL CHAKRA

MULADHARA

THE ROOT CHAKRA

HOW DOES ENERGY FLOW?

Our central nervous system controls most functions of the body and mind and is composed of our brain and our spinal cord, with the latter serving as the conduit for signals between the brain and the rest of the body. The chakra system of self-care teaches us that the energy flows along the spine and shows us the powerful connection between our mind and body and the important role the mind plays in our physical health.

Sushumna is the Sanskrit name for the central nadi, the dominant river of energy that flows through the body, running through the spinal cord and each of the seven chakras, to the brain. The word comes from sukha, meaning "joyful," and mana, meaning "mind." Our mind activates the parasympathetic nervous system, which is essential to maintain balance and harmony, as well as our sympathetic nervous system, which commands the fight-or-flight stimulant response. The parasympathetic nervous system is deeply connected to the chakra system, as it lies within the energetic points in the body that correlate with the chakras.

Our bodies are complex operating systems, but they have a simple objective: to maintain homeostasis, or a balanced internal state that allows for optimum functioning. Just as the sympathetic and parasympathetic nervous systems work together to help us perform energetic feats when needed, and to restore peaceful energetic states in order to maintain a harmonious balance, other parts of our bodies also work to maintain homeostasis.

As human beings on this earth, we will naturally experience energy blocks, stagnation, and imbalance. It is an unavoidable part of life. Since everything has energy, everything and anything can influence our energy positively or negatively. Emotions and thoughts are also energy, so what we think and feel has a huge influence on our energy bodies as well as our physical bodies.

When we have negative or repressed emotions or harmful thoughts, beliefs, and memories, these affect our energy bodies by causing blocks or stagnation. The source may be from a long-standing psychological issue stemming from childhood, an inherited fear or trauma from our parents, a major life event, or sometimes just getting stuck in really bad traffic—everything we experience impacts our energy. In turn, this can affect our physical health, resulting in all sorts of illnesses. While modern medicine is undoubtedly essential to our well-being, it often fails to deal with the root cause of sickness.

In order to be in a truly balanced state of health, we need to remove energetic and emotional toxins. You may be wondering how we do this, or whether it is even doable. The answer is that it's easier and more fun than you may think! Simple routines and rituals are such effective ways of maintaining energy flow. Daily life often throws energetic curveballs, so we simply need to counter them with routines and rituals that either serve as preventative measures to preserve our energy or counteract those disruptors to bring us back to a state of energetic equilibrium.

DIVINE FEMININE ENERGY

You may have heard the term *divine feminine* being referred to as a spiritual concept, and perhaps you think of this as some type of New Age jargon or as something that applies exclusively to females. In truth, the divine feminine energy is nothing new. It has always existed and has been acknowledged by different cultures in everything from religious and spiritual texts to art and literature.

As the name suggests, divine feminine energy represents what are traditionally thought of as more feminine qualities, such as being nurturing, intuitive, empathetic, and creative. This energy relates more to the right brain (intuition and emotions, often referred to as the feminine yin energy) versus the left (logic and analysis, often referred to as the masculine yang energy). In order to connect both and harness this energy, we need to engage in more gentle and nurturing activities that help us connect to our intuition and emotions, as well as feel connected to others, to planet Earth, and to Mother Nature herself.

This divine feminine energy plays an important role in each of our lives, regardless of gender, and is crucial to the healthy functioning of the world as a whole. Now more than ever before, our world needs the energy of nurturing, compassion, empathy, and love. As each of us awakens it within ourselves, so too can we awaken it externally for the world at large. We can harness chakra self-care to mindfully connect with our innate essence in order to harness divine feminine energy. We will discuss exactly how to do this later in the book as we explore each chakra.

REACHING KUNDALINI

Kundalini is a Sanskrit term for a dormant energy coiled at the base of the spine since birth. It is the source of prana. When kundalini awakens, the energy uncoils and flows freely up through the chakras, leading to an expanded state of consciousness, or bliss! This is the ultimate goal of chakra work: to connect and free the pure and powerful energy, which we were all born with, so it can flow freely through us and lead us to an expansion of bliss both internally (our consciousness) and externally (our bodies and lives). While awakening kundalini is a significant step in energetic healing and spiritual evolution, adjusting to the changes it can bring physically, emotionally, spiritually, and energetically can be disruptive. We must be patient with ourselves as we go through the process of healing our chakras, reaching kundalini, and integrating this new energy.

GETTING STARTED

As you embark on your healing journey, it is important to have the right environment in which to do the sacred work, which requires a special space and perhaps even an altar. Remember everything is about energy! In this space, you'll dive deep into journaling, meditating, and performing some rituals, all of which will allow you to connect to your higher self.

YOUR SACRED HEALING SPACE

Your sacred space provides both physical and energetic space and is essential to your healing journey. Think of it as a spiritual office of sorts, a space that is unique to you, feels safe and comfortable, and is peaceful and uplifting. To create this space, you don't need an entirely new room. You simply need a place where you can be comfortable and have a degree of privacy. This can be a corner of a room or a little nook. Walk around your home and find a place that feels good to you. And remember, it doesn't have to already be set up to be a sacred space—you can make it one! Incorporating nature in some way is always helpful to the energy of a sacred space, so perhaps the space can be by a window where natural light and fresh air flood in or even on a balcony or terrace where you can sit with the elements of Mother Nature (weather permitting!).

Wherever you choose to set up your space, make it only for the purposes of this work. It should be clean, tidy, and comfortable. As well as performing rituals, you will be writing and meditating there, so you will need to be able to sit and/or lie down comfortably. Perhaps this means a comfortable chair and desk setup, or maybe you can place lots of cushions or a beanbag on the floor to get cozy. You can be creative with your setup as long as it suits you.

In addition to a seating and writing arrangement, you will need some basic items: a dedicated journal and pen, candles, a candle snuffer, a white sage bundle, a palo santo stick, matchsticks or a lighter for your smudging rituals, crystals, and essential oils (we will discuss these in more detail as we go through each chakra).

☸ SMUDGING RITUAL

Burning sage is known as smudging, and this is a ritual that our ancestors used to help clear negative energy within a space or body or to assist in prayer or ritual. Sage is a woody herb that has a rich history of both medicinal and culinary uses and has been renowned across cultures and countries around the world for its healing properties for thousands of years.

Smudging has become a popular practice to both clear unwanted energies and help positive energy flow. When sage burns, negative ions are released into the air. Contrary to what the term suggests, negative ions actually increase our sense of well-being and improve our mental state, thus bringing more positivity into our lives. Before you begin any of the rituals in this book, you will normally have to smudge.

Before you begin smudging, set an intention of what you wish to achieve. Is it to clear negative energy within a space, yourself, or an object? Is it to bring more energetic balance and calm? Or is it to relax you or prepare you for another ritual or meditation? Come ready with this intention before you commence the Smudging Ritual.

1. Close all the windows and make sure no fan or air conditioner is on.
2. Take a few deep breaths in and out, and set your intention.

3. Light a sage bundle or a few leaves of a sage bundle. Gently blow on it.

4. Wave the sage gently around yourself, the object, or the space you are purifying. If you are clearing a space, take the sage and wave it into each corner of the area, from floor to ceiling, tracing the entire space and making sure to get into every nook and cranny. You can use a small cup or dish underneath the sage to catch any burning embers.

5. As you wave the sage in the appropriate places, come back to your intention and visualize it as you see the smoke rise from the sage.

6. Once you are finished, you can open a window to let in fresh air.

7. To seal the Smudging Ritual, you can light sweet incense or a candle, diffuse a floral essential oil (e.g., jasmine), or spray rosewater around yourself or the space. This brings a sweet and light energy into the purified space.

SACRED ALTAR

In your sacred space, you can create a personal altar. Altars are used by people of many different religions and traditions, and can be found in many places of worship. However, altars transcend religion and, in fact, are increasingly popular in people's homes as a powerful personal tool for spiritual connection. If you choose to make one, your altar will serve as a special tool for your individual spiritual connection and healing journey.

Setting up an altar is actually a simple, fun, and creative process. The physical item you use as your altar depends on the furniture you have available and the space in your home. It can be anything from a corner or an end table to a cabinet, counter, nightstand, or wall shelf. There is no right or wrong object. Use what works for you given your space and what feels good.

Once you've decided what you will use for your altar, you can choose what to include on it. Sacred items connected to nature and the four elements should be placed on your altar. You can include candles (fire), incense (air), sand or dirt (earth), or a little pot of water or a water feature (water). Other items to include are crystals, plants, statues, shells, feathers, and so on. These are just a few examples. There is no limit to the tools and items you can include on your altar. Personalize it to suit you.

Once you have chosen your altar and sacred tools, you need to cleanse them because, as we know, everything has energy and there may be certain energies you don't want to bring into your sacred space. You can use the sage bundle to perform a Smudging Ritual during which you burn the smoke around the items with the intention of cleansing them of any low vibrational, or negative, energies.

COLLECTING CRYSTALS

Crystals are stones or rocks made of minerals found on Earth. They have natural healing energies. There are many different types of crystals that offer different properties, depending on which geological formation they were formed in.

For the purposes of our work in this book, you will need to get a few crystals, ideally one for each chakra. (In forthcoming chapters, I offer recommendations for chakra stones, but you can make do with just one for each chakra.) Polished stones are best because, as you will see, you will often use these crystals in massage and meditation, so you want ones without sharp edges! I also highly recommend buying a couple of crystal wands, such as selenite and quartz wands, as you can use these for multiple chakras and for general energy-balancing work, in ritual and meditation.

There is no right or wrong way to buy crystals, but it is important to buy ones you feel connected to in some way. Don't overthink this. It can be as simple as liking the color or shape of a particular stone. Although it is fun to go crystal shopping and pick up stones to get a feel for them, it is just as fun to get the perfect crystals online. Some of my favorite crystals are ones I purchased over the internet! No matter where you buy your crystals, make sure to conduct a smudging ceremony to clear the energy around them before you begin using them.

HEALTHY EXPECTATIONS

Just like snowflakes, we are all intricately unique, and where each of us finds ourselves today is a different energetic place than our neighbor. As you start your chakra journey, remember this is your journey of healing, alignment, and self-care, and thus will be unique to you. Be kind and patient with yourself as you go through this process, and try not to deem it unsuccessful just because you aren't seeing immediate progress. Remember, you are peeling back and reconfiguring years of energy. There isn't a right or wrong length of time to achieve a milestone. Your journey to optimum energetic well-being will take as long as it needs to.

In addition, as we progress on our path of healing, we may need assistance in clearing energetic blocks and imbalances. Whether it's a hands-on healing treatment by a Reiki healer, or energy healer, or a session where we talk through emotional matters with a therapist or spiritual teacher or mentor, getting a helping hand (or ear!) is sometimes just what the universe ordered for us to make progress along our path. I say this from personal experience, as I saw a number of different energy healers and had countless sessions over the years. Not only did this help me on my personal path to healing, but it also inspired me to train and become a healer myself. My healers became my teachers and allowed me to heal others and, in time, to train others as healers! So I know from personal experience the many healing modalities, practitioners, and teachers that can support and guide you on your journey to energetic alignment. Be open to getting help on your healing path, and take time to find an experienced and reputable practitioner whom you feel aligned with.

USING ESSENTIAL OILS

Essential oils are often used in aromatherapy, a form of alternative healing that uses plant extracts and scents to help with certain ailments and support well-being. These oils can be inhaled directly, used in an oil diffuser, or dabbed onto the skin (directly or diluted, depending on the oil). You can also combine different ones to make your own custom oil blend, which is one of my favorite ways to work with essential oils.

Throughout the book, I make essential oil recommendations for each chakra and explain the properties of these oils and why they will assist that particular energy center. I'll also provide you with oil blend recipes to try out for each chakra. Just as with the crystals, you don't need to purchase multiple essential oils for each chakra—simply start with one for each.

As you learn about the different essential oils recommended for each of the chakras, notice if you feel called to one more than another. You will also notice that some essential oils work for multiple chakras. Perhaps you already know the scent of some of the oils and enjoy them. That's a sure sign that you will benefit from those oils! If possible, find a local store that sells essential oils and sniff them to see what you like or what feels good. Follow your nose!

CHAKRA CHECK-IN

Now it is time to check in and see how your energy centers are functioning as we embark on the process of identifying and healing any energetic imbalances. Please know that this meditative check-in is to help you connect to your energy body and conduct an overall checkup as to how it is functioning. As we delve into each chakra in depth, you will get custom meditations to help connect to that specific chakra and balance and heal it. So, think of this initial chakra check-in as the start of connecting and consciously working with your energy body.

1. Carve out some quiet time in your sacred space. Smudge your space to clear the energy (see the Smudging Ritual on p. 19).

2. Find a comfortable position to either sit or lie down for the duration of this meditation (around 15 minutes). Close your eyes, then take a few deep breaths in and out of your nose to help your mind focus and settle your heart rate.

3. Set the intention: This is the start of connecting with your energetic body. Invite in divine guidance, whether from God, angels, your ancestors, departed loved ones, the universe, or simply your own intuition.

4. Begin the process of "scanning" your body at each chakra, starting from the soles of your feet and moving up to your lower back, then your lower abdomen (around two inches below your belly button), then your midsection around your belly button, moving up to your chest, your neck, and then the space between your eyebrows and your forehead, finally finishing with the crown of your head. At each chakra, think about each part of your body. Try your best not to overthink this process, but rather just observe what you may sense, see, or feel as you move through each chakra. Ask yourself:

- What does it feel like?

- What can I see? You might see a color, a shape, or an image. Or perhaps you will envision a memory, an emotion, or a feeling.

5. After you finish this process, thank your energy body for this connection and then gently open your eyes. Write down as many of your observations as you can recall. Don't worry if they don't make sense; just make a note of them.

6. Light a candle, drink herbal tea, and take some time to reflect upon your meditation and journal any insights. Try not to analyze what you felt, but write freely instead. Here are some prompts to consider:

- How do you generally feel about the state of your energetic body?

- Does it feel light and free-flowing, or heavy and constricted?

- How does each area/chakra feel?

- Do you feel any are imbalanced or blocked in some way?

- Is there physical tension?

This exercise should give you insight into your energy body: how each chakra is currently operating and which chakras may need more help. Next, we will discuss each chakra in depth, including what each chakra governs; symptoms of imbalance; and how to open, balance, and heal each chakra so its energy flows optimally. You can also jump ahead to the chapters on the chakras you are most interested in and focus on those parts right away.

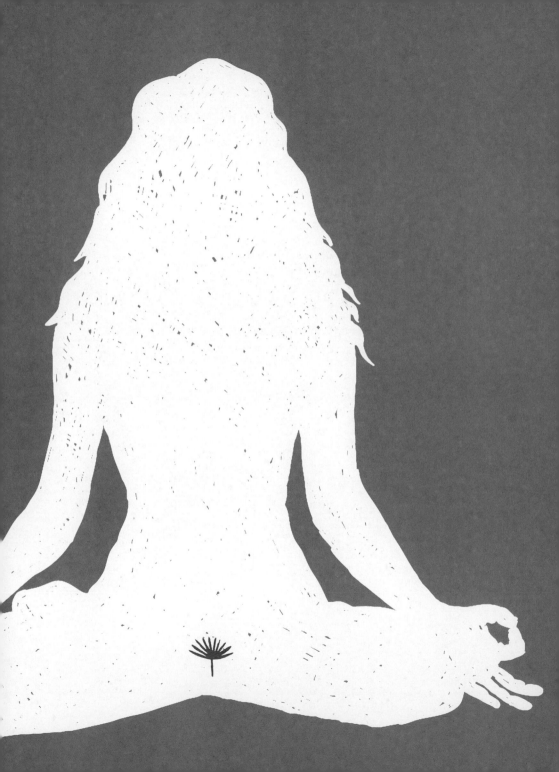

TWO

ROOT CHAKRA

WHEN THE ROOT IS DEEP,
THERE IS NO REASON TO
FEAR THE WIND.

Unknown

As the first of the chakras, the root chakra is the foundation of all the other chakras and is the lowest, found at the base of the spine, just below the tailbone. It is also the first of what are known as the lower chakras, comprising the root, sacral, and solar plexus. The Sanskrit name for this chakra is Muladhara, which means "root" (mula) and "existence" (adhara). It is from this translation that the foundational chakra has become more commonly known as the "root" or "base" chakra.

The root chakra governs the foundations of our lives and core issues, including our basic needs, sense of security, our home and family life, and how we feel in our bodies and on this earth. These aspects of life are our roots; they help us to be grounded and to not only survive but also thrive. The energy of our root chakra determines our ability to be firmly rooted within ourselves and the world.

When the root chakra is functioning optimally and is in healthy alignment, we have an inner sense of security, which manifests as clear thinking and good concentration, which allows us to set goals and prioritize and carry out tasks in order to achieve those goals. A healthy, balanced root chakra lends to a calm, steady, and graceful energy that we can harness to remain grounded yet flexible during transitional periods, and to be resourceful and courageous during more challenging times. In this sense, the healthy and aligned energy of the root chakra helps energetically fuel our lives in all areas, including what we manifest and how we navigate our path during both highs and lows.

ROOT CHAKRA IMBALANCE

When the root chakra energies are either imbalanced or blocked in some way, we are impacted both emotionally and physically, which in turn influences aspects of our lives. It is important to note that an unbalanced chakra can be either underactive or overactive. When the root chakra is underactive, that means it is closed in some way. As a result, we may feel restless, lethargic, anxious and panicky, frustrated or angry, resentful, and disconnected from both ourselves and the world. As a result, we may have low self-esteem and feel pessimistic, insecure, unsafe, and as though we don't fit in. This often

CORRESPONDENCES

COLOR	ELEMENT	SYMBOL	SHAPE
Red	Earth		Cube

PLANETS

Earth   Saturn

ASTROLOGICAL SIGN

Capricorn

STONES

Red tiger's eye   Hematite

Garnet   Smoky quartz

Bloodstone

GODDESS ARCHETYPE

The Goddess Mother

ANIMAL

Elephant

ESSENTIAL OILS

Vetiver   Patchouli

Lavender   Frankincense

Sandalwood

manifests as feeling overwhelmed and disorganized, finding it hard to focus on even the simplest of tasks, and being ungrounded in our physical realities.

If the root chakra is overactive, it is almost as though energy is working overtime. In this case, we may get annoyed or even angry and aggressive at the slightest provocation. We can find ourselves too attached to the physical and material world and therefore over-indulge in money, food, sex, and so on. We may be overly rooted and fixed in our position—in other words, resistant to change and obsessed with feeling secure all the time.

As our root chakra literally relates to our roots, it can be negatively impacted by unresolved events from our childhood that made us feel unsafe or insecure, which results in the root chakra being imbalanced. As the wheels of life turn, the root chakra can also easily become blocked or imbalanced by events that threaten our sense of basic security. Whether these are real-life events or perceived threats, they all act to disrupt the flow of the root chakra. For example, insecurity regarding a relationship or job ignites fear, impacting the healthy, aligned flow of the root chakra.

The root chakra governs the adrenal glands, bladder, kidneys, lower extremities, and spine. When this chakra is imbalanced, you can experience physical symptoms that include the following:

- Constipation
- Weight issues

- Digestive issues
- An eating disorder (over- or undereating)
- Fatigue/lethargy
- Back pain
- Increased anxiety (including panic attacks or similar symptoms)
- Feeling unsafe
- Negativity and/or pessimism
- Difficulty concentrating
- Low self-esteem
- Clumsiness

WHEN THE ROOT CHAKRA OPENS

As the root chakra opens and falls into alignment, we may feel heat in our lower back and a tingling sensation as previously blocked energy starts to flow again. This can result in the feeling of vibrations across our entire body as the root chakra moves energy to all parts of our physical being. We may experience certain cravings or a shift in appetite in order for us to feel more grounded within our bodies and the planet. Common sensations of an opened root chakra are feeling one's feet more and feeling heavier, both of which are actually a result of our being more in our bodies and grounded in the earth.

Sometimes during the process of opening and balancing this chakra, we may experience a reappearance of prior ailments from when it was out of alignment. On a physical level, these can range from aches and pains to digestive issues, fatigue, and even insomnia. Emotional issues related to a blocked root chakra may temporarily resurface and/or become exacerbated. This can be distressing, as you may feel as though you are taking one step forward only to take two back; however, this is actually part of the important healing process of rebalancing this foundational chakra. Rest assured; these feelings are temporary.

GODDESS ARCHETYPE: THE GODDESS MOTHER

The root chakra connects to the Goddess Mother archetype. This archetype, like the divine feminine energy, transcends gender, as it represents nurturing energy that anyone can have. The Goddess Mother feeds, nourishes, and provides for our needs. She is compassionate and loving, full of encouragement and optimism, and is a positive force in our lives. Her energy is given to us to sustain ourselves physically and emotionally.

Some of the names and figures in history associated with the Goddess Mother are the Virgin Mary, Venus, and Quan Yin. The most ancient and powerful of these Goddess Mothers are Mother Nature and Earth herself, often referred to as Gaia, the mother to us all, who sustains our very existence. The names of the Goddess Mother have changed as mankind has evolved, but her basic persona as the bearer and guardian of all life remains.

When we apply the traits of the Goddess Mother to the function of the foundational chakra, we are reminded of the mothering, nurturing role of the root chakra. It helps us to feel secure and safe, providing a strong foundation from which we are able to flourish.

When you become your own Goddess Mother, you take responsibility for your circumstances and are able to manage the curveballs life throws at you. Eating well, getting enough rest, and becoming less reliant on others are ways to help develop the Goddess Mother archetype in you. Mothering and nourishing yourself means understanding what you need and then providing that for yourself, to the best of your ability. The more we can adopt the traits of the Goddess Mother, the healthier and more stable we become.

On a personal level, the Goddess Mother was among my favorite archetypes to work with on my journey of healing and alignment, and is the one I resonate most deeply with.

ROOT CHAKRA STONES

The crystals associated with the root chakra tend to be darker in color, evoking earth energies and helping us to ground ourselves. Each crystal has unique properties to heal and balance the root chakra.

RED TIGER'S EYE

Use red tiger's eye to overcome lethargy, which can be present with an imbalanced root chakra. This stone helps with motivating a sense of joie de vivre, or "zest for life." It can be used to clarify and amplify the energies of the root chakra and, in turn, assist all the other chakras. I like to hold a few small polished red tiger's eye stones during meditation or keep some nearby during times when I feel my root chakra is imbalanced.

GARNET

Red or earthy brown, garnet is a powerfully grounding yet energizing stone. It can be used in challenging situations, as it helps us to be courageous and hopeful, thus boosting our natural survival instincts. A raw garnet is beautiful and powerful. It's useful to have on your altar and to keep nearby during meditation.

BLOODSTONE

Used in ancient Babylon, bloodstone was considered to be magical. It's a powerful healer and revitalizer with grounding and protective energies. It helps mitigate some of the symptoms of an overactive root chakra, such as irritability, impatience, and anger. A large polished bloodstone is very useful for meditation and ritual. You can hold it in your hands, place it on your root chakra, or use it to massage essential oils into this energy center.

HEMATITE

This nearly all-black stone helps harmonize the mind, body, and soul by removing excess energy and separating your emotions from the emotions of others, thus grounding you in your own reality and enhancing your pure personal energy. This stone dissolves negativity, restores balance, and acts as a protector. I love using hematite wands after healing sessions. In rituals, I shower or bathe and meditate with a hematite wand in each hand (a surefire way to release any energy that does not belong to me). I highly recommend hematite wands for any empaths.

SMOKY QUARTZ

Smoky quartz is one of the most efficient grounding and cleansing crystals. It serves as a protective stone, acting as a stress reliever by connecting you to the earth. It can absorb and transmute significant amounts of negative energy and release it into the earth to be neutralized naturally. It provides a vital shield against mental, emotional, and environmental stressors. A smoky quartz wand is a must in your crystal collection, as you can use it for healing, for meditation and ritual, and to amplify the energies of your other stones.

ROOT CHAKRA ESSENTIAL OILS

The recommended oils for the root chakra have earthy, calming, and grounding properties that promote peace of mind and balance.

FRANKINCENSE

For thousands of years, frankincense oil has been used for spiritual purposes and considered holy oil. It comes from tree resin, thus connecting us to the physical world. It is a very soothing and grounding oil that can take the edge off racing thoughts and restlessness. Diffusing this oil can immediately shift the energy in your space or within you to a more tranquil state. I recommend it for your essential oil collection.

SANDALWOOD

Sandalwood comes from the Santalum tree, and its scent can relieve anxiety and irritability. This oil is wonderful for calming emotional stress and helps promote a sense of inner peace. It is often diffused and used in meditation or yoga classes to help energetically assist those attending. A few direct inhalations of sandalwood oil before bed can aid with having a restful night of sleep.

VETIVER

Vetiver oil is very powerful in soothing the nervous system thanks to its calming and grounding properties. Rub this oil into the soles of your feet or the small of your back before meditating or going to bed at night.

LAVENDER

One of the most popular and well-known relaxing and stress-relieving oils is lavender. As well as diffusing this oil to instantly create a peaceful environment, you can combine it with other oils to bring even more tranquility to yourself and your environment.

PATCHOULI

This healing oil comes from the patchouli plant. It is effective at relieving constipation, which is a symptom of an underactive root chakra. Massage it into your lower back and around your belly first thing in the morning to help your digestive tract.

PEACE OF MIND BLEND

This root chakra oil blend will help you be grounded and relaxed, bringing you to a state of inner peace and confidence. You can use your daily blend as part of a ritual or meditation, as a massage oil, or as a stabilizing fragrance by gently rubbing it on your wrists or temples.

INGREDIENTS

2 tbsp	jojoba oil (or another carrier oil of your choice)
3 drops	sandalwood essential oil
3 drops	vetiver essential oil
2 drops	frankincense essential oil
1 drop	patchouli essential oil

TOOLS/EQUIPMENT

2 oz. dark glass bottle
Dropper

YIELD

Makes 1.5 oz.

1. Pour the jojoba oil into a dark glass bottle.

2. Using a dropper, add each essential oil. Cover the bottle and swirl lightly.

3. Massage the oil onto your lower back, the soles of your feet, your temples, or wrists, as needed. (For external use only.)

◇ ROOT CHAKRA VISUALIZATION

Before you begin this meditation, smudge using a white sage bundle or palo santo to clear the energy. Then either diffuse sandalwood oil or light sandalwood incense, light a candle, and turn off any lights for ambiance.

1. Lie down and close your eyes.
2. Take a deep breath in through your nose, exhale out through your mouth, and sigh. Let your muscles soften and your body relax. Repeat this as many times as needed until you feel relaxed and ready for meditation.
3. As you continue to inhale and exhale deeply, visualize your breath coming in and out of the base of your spine.
4. Keeping your eyes closed, repeat to yourself (either silently or aloud), "I acknowledge and honor my root chakra, and so I see it clearly."
5. Visualize a red cube at the base of your spine. Look at the color and size of this cube. Observe its corners and points as well as any other details, like if it is spinning or static. Notice how this cube feels and what insights you receive about any imbalances or blockages and what you may need to do in order to bring the root chakra to energetic equilibrium.

6. Once you have observed the cube and obtained sufficient insight into the functioning of your root chakra, take a moment to acknowledge and give gratitude to this energy point in your body, and then gently open your eyes.

✿ ROOT CHAKRA ACTIVATION

Before you begin this activation exercise, cleanse your sacred space by smudging, and also cleanse yourself by smudging around your body from the top of your head to the bottom of your feet. Light a grounding incense stick, such as frankincense or sandalwood, or diffuse a root chakra essential oil. You should also be barefoot for this exercise, but you can wear socks for warmth if needed.

1. Begin in a standing position, but if necessary, you can sit on a chair. Stand (or sit) tall, and imagine there is an invisible cord at the top of your head that is pulling you up. Allow this cord to help lift your head, in turn straightening your spine and neck but keeping your shoulders low and dropped.

2. Bring your attention to your feet and really plant them on the ground, visualizing that there are tree roots growing out of the soles of your feet and into the earth.

3. Now focus on your lower back, and visualize the red cube that represents your root chakra, which you identified in the visualization meditation. Start to expand this cube, seeing it become larger and brighter and more alive. See it turning in a clockwise direction, starting slowly and picking up speed until it is spinning fully and freely. Visualize the energy flowing from this red cube and your root chakra throughout your body. You can visualize this as a reddish-brown light that permeates your entire physical being.

4. As you sense this energy flooding your body, feel a deep sense of gratitude for the healthy functioning of this energy center. Gently open your eyes when you are finished.

❀ ROOT CHAKRA REFLECTION

Make yourself a cup of tea, ideally decaffeinated and earthy, such as rooibos or dandelion. Diffuse the root chakra essential oils, and gather your journal and a smooth wand, either hematite or smoky quartz (or both), which you can hold in one hand or place nearby. You can write in your sacred space or find an outdoor space. Nature may prove very powerful, given this exercise is for the root chakra.

Reflect on your experiences of the Root Chakra Visualization and Activation. Think back to the scenarios and traits associated with either an imbalanced or blocked root chakra, which we identified earlier. Note if you have any insights that may help you understand what you need to do in order for this chakra to be balanced and spinning freely. Here are some questions to ask yourself:

- Do you get annoyed or agitated easily?
- How stable are the foundations of your life?
- How secure do you feel about your home life, work life, and finances?
- How easily do you deal with sudden change?
- Do you avoid change, even if it could be positive, because you are fearful of it?
- Do you feel you deserve the things you want in life?
- Do you have perseverance when striving for your goals?
- Do you feel supported in manifesting your goals? By whom are you supported: a spirit, God, a divine force, or the universe?

ROOT CHAKRA AFFIRMATIONS

Stating affirmations, or mantras, will help you to connect to the traits of an open, healthy, flowing root chakra. They will help you connect to your inner strength and have faith in your ability to withstand the ebb and flow of life. You can do this exercise by speaking the affirmations to yourself or to your mirrored reflection in a space that feels sacred to you. Do this exercise daily, ideally in the morning and at night, as you go through the process of opening and balancing the root chakra. During transitional or more challenging times, you can do this multiple times a day and can also repeat the mantra silently if you don't feel comfortable speaking it out loud. Here are some affirmations you can say in your head or out loud:

- I am centered and balanced.
- From this strong inner foundation, I know I can handle any situation that comes my way.
- I trust in the process of life with all its peaks and valleys.
- I have the courage and strength to manifest the life of my dreams.
- I know I deserve all that is good.
- I nurture myself, and life nurtures me.
- I am optimistic and focused.
- I have faith in myself and my abilities.
- I trust that I am divinely guided by the universe every day.
- I trust that I have all that I need internally to create all I desire externally.
- I am a channel for peace and serenity.
- I choose peace and calm.

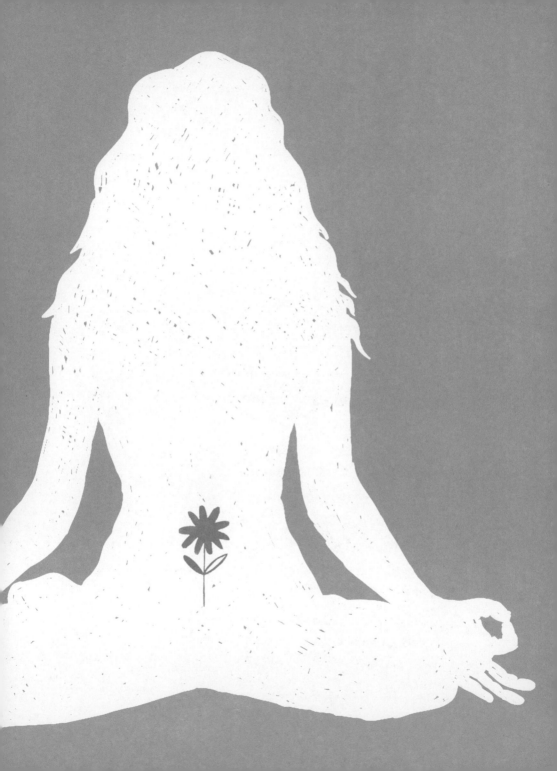

THREE

SACRAL CHAKRA

PASSION IS ENERGY.
FEEL THE POWER THAT
COMES FROM FOCUSING
ON WHAT EXCITES YOU.

Oprah Winfrey

The sacral is the second of the chakras and is found in the lower abdomen, just below the navel and above the pubic bone. The Sanskrit name for the sacral chakra is Swadhisthana, made up of two Sanskrit words—swa, meaning "one's own," and adhisthana, meaning "abode or dwelling place." *Sacral* relates to the anatomical area by the sacrum, and it also means "holy" or "sacred." So, it is fitting that this chakra houses our emotions, passions, and pleasures—the things that emotionally satiate us and give us joy, and so are sacred to us.

This chakra is considered to be the creative and sexual energy center of our bodies and is thus linked to matters of intimacy and connection, including sex, fertility, and reproduction. When the sacral chakra is functioning optimally, we are content, uninhibited in our relationships and creative endeavors, and capable of deep intimacy, and we exude a joyful vibrancy.

SACRAL CHAKRA IMBALANCE

As this chakra is about our emotional health, an imbalance can interfere with enjoying life. If the sacral chakra energies are stuck, stagnant, or blocked in some way, we will be impacted both emotionally and physically, which in turn will influence the creative and sexual aspects of our lives.

With an underactive sacral chakra, we are likely to suffer from a low libido, issues around sex or intimacy, gynecological or fertility challenges, struggles with creative endeavors, a lack of creative insights or fulfillment, lingering relationship issues, and emotional dissatisfaction. Conversely, if the sacral chakra is overactive, this can manifest as overwhelming emotions, mood swings, excessive highs and lows, dramatic situations in relationships, overdependence on others, jealousy and possessiveness, and sexual or other addictions.

Our sacral chakra can be impacted by energetic baggage we carry over from our root chakra, which can prevent us from feeling safe to experience joy. Perhaps this is from our childhood and family, or communal or societal conditioning around self-expression, sex and sexuality—or even just general enjoyment of life. As we navigate each day, circumstances like relationship issues, sexual experiences, and how we handle our work–life balance may also disrupt the flow of this chakra.

CORRESPONDENCES

COLOR	ELEMENT	SYMBOL	SHAPE
Orange	Water		Pyramid

PLANET

Jupiter

ASTROLOGICAL SIGNS

Cancer   Scorpio

STONES

Carnelian
Onyx
Orange spinel

GODDESS ARCHETYPE

The Goddess
Empress

ANIMAL

Crocodile

ESSENTIAL OILS

Rosewood   Clary sage
Ylang-ylang   Orange

The sacral chakra governs the sexual organs, liver, hormones, upper intestines, and spleen. When this chakra is imbalanced, you may experience symptoms such as the following:

- Sexual dysfunction
- Low libido
- Sexual addictions
- Addictions to substances (drugs, alcohol, etc.)
- Pelvic pain
- Hormonal issues
- Fertility challenges
- Urinary issues
- Sciatica/lower back pain
- Guilt
- Emotional imbalances
- Mood disorders
- Lack of fulfilment and joy
- Boredom
- Dissatisfaction

WHEN THE SACRAL CHAKRA OPENS

As the sacral chakra opens and aligns, you may feel a warm tingling or vibration in your lower abdomen as energy starts to flow fully. This can result in changes in our digestive system as well as hormonal and reproductive shifts. Your libido may awaken, and you may find yourself more sexually aroused. Fertility issues caused by prior hormonal imbalances can improve. You may take more pleasure in everyday activities, such as eating and drinking, and feel more inclined to participate in hobbies and other pleasurable pursuits. You may have a creative awakening and feel inspired.

At first, as with any of the chakras, you may also experience a healing crisis of sorts during the integration and alignment of the sacral chakra energies. Physically, this may manifest as lower back or pelvic pain, urinary tract infections, or even a resurgence or temporary worsening of hormonal or reproductive issues. You may even go through an emotional purge of sorts, but this is purely so you can reset emotionally and become more balanced and joyful. Be patient with yourself as this healing and alignment takes place, and know that joy awaits on the other side of this process.

GODDESS ARCHETYPE: THE GODDESS EMPRESS

The Goddess Empress is the archetype of the sacral chakra. She enjoys all the physical aspects of life on Earth. She knows that she deserves to experience pleasure and joy, so she is passionate and satiated by life. She is in touch with her body and her sexuality. Sensual and soft, she feels deeply but is emotionally balanced and has an air of graceful serenity about her. She trusts that there is always more than enough and, as a result, is generous and giving. Her energy and appetite for life draw others to her.

Famous queens and empresses have been associated with the Goddess Empress archetype, including Empress Wu Zetian of China and the Queen of Sheba, a powerful ruler of ancient Ethiopia who enchanted King Solomon with her beauty and generous, joyful spirit.

When we infuse the energies of the Goddess Empress into our sacral chakra, we remember that joy is our divine birthright, and so we allow ourselves to experience pleasures of all sorts. Joy and peace become our emotional foundation, which not only makes us charismatic to others but also attracts good fortune. We are open channels for creativity and relish the process of birthing new ideas. Adopting the Goddess Empress helps us remember that we deserve the good things in life, which in turn magnetizes us to attract those things to us.

SACRAL CHAKRA STONES

Many of the recommended stones for the sacral chakra have revitalizing and vibrant energies and come in the color of the chakra.

ORANGE CALCITE

Orange calcite is deeply cleansing and energizing. This gem helps balance emotions and removes fear that may be stored in the energy body. It is also known as the creativity stone.

CARNELIAN

A stabilizing stone, carnelian helps restore vitality and can boost one's zest for life. Often used for meditation, it can calm emotions such as anger, jealousy, and envy. By clearing the mind of unnecessary thoughts, this stone helps bring clarity and peace of mind.

ORANGE SPINEL

In Reiki, orange spinel is known for opening and aligning the sacral chakra. Holding this stone or using it in meditation can help us tap into our intuition and stimulate creativity. Many healing practitioners call this stone the fertility stone. I recommend using this powerful healing stone in polished form on the body.

ONYX

Onyx is a black stone that is excellent at absorbing and transforming negativity. It also helps us release mental, physical, and spiritual blockages that may be preventing us from experiencing joy and creativity. Polished onyx stones are highly effective for healing rituals, meditation, and chakra balancing.

SACRAL CHAKRA ESSENTIAL OILS

These essential oils have properties that aid in the healthy functioning of the sacral chakra. Many are quite sweet and uplifting, which promotes the vibrant nature of the second chakra.

ROSEWOOD

Extracted from the rosewood tree, this oil has a floral yet woodsy aroma. It is known for its aphrodisiac qualities and can also help calm an overworked mind, helping to restore emotional balance. Dab a few drops on your temples and gently massage them in to bring more harmony and peace of mind. You can also use it with a carrier oil for self-massage, or with a partner, to help stimulate the sacral chakra.

YLANG-YLANG

This feel-good oil promotes a sense of joy and happiness, whether diffused or used in a blend for massage or moisturizing. With its sweet, romantic aroma, ylang-ylang is the most renowned aphrodisiac oil and can also be worn as an oil perfume.

CLARY SAGE

One of the best essential oils for the female reproductive system, clary sage treats menstrual issues, such as cramps and premenstrual tension, and can help regulate the menstrual cycle and hormones. Clary sage became one of my must-have essential oils after I found that massaging a few drops directly on my lower abdomen alleviated the pain of menstrual cramps.

ORANGE

Orange oil is one of the most uplifting oils. Diffusing it can create a joyful environment, which is so helpful for activating the vibrant energy of the sacral chakra. The aroma allows us to think positively and feel happy, and it stimulates creativity.

JOYFUL CREATION BLEND

The sacral chakra custom oil blend is designed to help you connect to your passion and creative nature. You can use this oil blend daily when going through the process of opening and aligning this energy center, or use it when you need to experience more of the traits of a healthily functioning sacral chakra. This oil is best sniffed directly or massaged gently into your lower abdomen and the sides of your neck. It makes for a great aphrodisiac!

INGREDIENTS

2 tbsp   rose hip oil
5 drops   rosewood essential oil
3 drops   ylang-ylang
          essential oil

TOOLS/EQUIPMENT

2 oz. dark glass bottle
Dropper

YIELD

Makes 1.5 oz.

1. Pour the rose hip oil into a dark glass bottle.

2. Using a dropper, add each essential oil. Cover the bottle and swirl lightly.

3. Massage gently into your lower abdomen around the sacral chakra. Use it also as an oil perfume by rubbing gently on your temples, wrists, and neck. (For external use only.)

ꕥ SACRAL CHAKRA VISUALIZATION

You can do this meditation on your bed or in your sacred space. Prepare by clearing the energy with a Smudging Ritual, using either a white sage bundle or a palo santo stick. You can then diffuse one of the recommended sacral chakra essential oils, perhaps even combining two of the oils. If you have some of the stones associated with the sacral chakra, collect them, as they will be useful for the meditation. Turn on a soft-focus lamp or light a candle for ambiance before lying down and getting comfortable.

1. Lie down and close your eyes.
2. Take a deep breath in through your nose, exhale out through your mouth, and sigh. Let your muscles soften and your body relax. Repeat this as many times as needed until you feel relaxed and ready for meditation.
3. Gently place your hands on the area below your belly button and above the pelvic bone. Continuing to inhale and exhale deeply, visualize your breath coming in through your hands and entering your lower abdomen as you exhale.
4. Keeping your eyes closed, repeat to yourself (either silently or aloud), "I honor and cherish my sacral chakra, and so I see it clearly."

5. Visualize an orange pyramid in your lower abdomen. Carefully observe the pyramid's elements. Notice if it has any details, including if it is spinning or static. Notice how this pyramid feels and what insights you receive about any imbalances or blockages and what you may need to do in order to bring your sacral chakra to energetic equilibrium.

6. Once you have observed the pyramid and obtained sufficient insight into the functioning of your sacral chakra, take a moment to acknowledge and give gratitude to this energy point in your body, and then gently open your eyes.

❁ SACRAL CHAKRA ACTIVATION

Before you begin this activation exercise, take a few minutes to conduct a smudging ceremony to clear the energy around your sacred space and yourself, and then diffuse orange or another sacral chakra oil of your choice. Massage a few drops of the Joyful Creation Blend (p. 55), ylang-ylang oil, or rosewood oil onto your lower abdomen.

1. Lie down, then take some of the sacral chakra stones and place them between your hands and abdomen.

2. Close your eyes and visualize an orange light emitting from your hands and entering your abdomen with your breath. See this orange light moving into your body, filling up your lower abdomen.

3. Bring your mind's eye to the orange pyramid, which represents your sacral chakra. See the orange light flowing from your hands and into your abdomen to fill the pyramid. As it is flooded with this bright orange light, the pyramid grows in stature and vibrancy and begins to spin in a clockwise direction, slowly picking up speed until the pyramid is moving so fast it now appears as a vivid orange light spinning in your lower abdomen and flooding the rest of your body with energy. As you see this vivid orange energy permeating your body, invite in a sense of joy and passion for yourself, others, and life.

🪷 SACRAL CHAKRA REFLECTION

Prepare some tea, perhaps an orange peel, lemongrass, and rose hip infusion. Get settled in your sacred space or another space that feels comfortable to you. Diffuse one or more of the sacral chakra oils and light a candle. Gently massage a few drops of the Joyful Creation Blend (p. 55) or orange oil onto your lower abdomen, temples, and wrists. Place some of the sacral chakra stones nearby, or hold some in one hand.

As you journal, reflect on your experiences of the Sacral Chakra Visualization and Activation. Consider what you learned about your sacral chakra and how an imbalanced or blocked sacral chakra may make you feel. Check in as to whether you are experiencing some of these symptoms. Note any insights you receive as to what you may need to do for this chakra to be open and balanced. Here are some questions to ask yourself as you reflect:

- Are you giving yourself free time to do fun things?
- Are you allowing yourself to indulge in treatments for your body, such as a facial, massage, or scrub?
- Do you feel you deserve to enjoy life?
- Are you able to see and experience joy and pleasure in the small things?

- Do you like your body, and are you comfortable and confident in it?
- Are you comfortable with your sexuality?
- Do you feel sensual?
- Do you feel abundant? Does life feel abundant to you?
- Are you involved in negative drama?

❀ SACRAL CHAKRA AFFIRMATIONS

Sacral chakra affirmations help connect you to your body and pleasure center, reminding you that you deserve to enjoy your body in this physical life! Say the mantras twice a day, as a morning and evening ritual, while you are in the process of opening and balancing the sacral chakra. Dab some of the Joyful Creation Blend (p. 55) or any of the other sacral chakra oils on your neck, wrists, temples, and lower abdomen before you begin. To best benefit from these affirmations, it is good to move your body when affirming the words. Ideally, do some form of yin activity, such as yoga or dance, really feeling what you are saying in your body. You can create your own mantras or use the suggestions below. As with all the mantras, you can also repeat them silently.

- I am a divinely created being, here to enjoy all that is divine in life.
- I know I deserve to experience pleasure, and I take pleasure in all of life.
- My body is sacred, and I cherish it.
- It is safe for me to express and enjoy my sexuality.
- I honor my feelings and am able to move through them in a healthy way.
- I allow myself time to create and play, just for the joy of it!
- I honor and enjoy my body.
- My sexuality is sacred.
- I feel pleasure every day.
- I am passionate about life.
- I am playful.
- I am joyful.
- I honor all of my emotions.
- Creativity flows through me.
- Joy flows through me.
- Abundance flows through me.

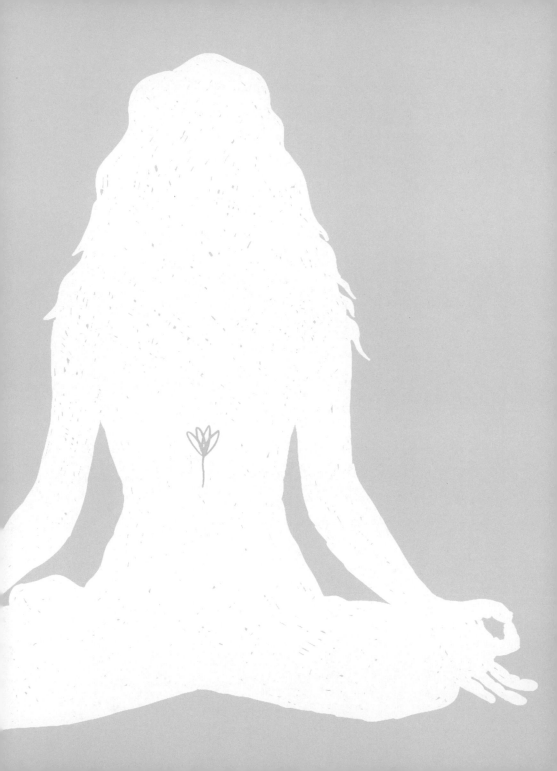

FOUR

SOLAR PLEXUS CHAKRA

**PERSONAL POWER IS THE
ABILITY TO TAKE ACTION.**

Tony Robbins

As the third of the chakras, the solar plexus chakra is the last in the trio of lower chakras. The Sanskrit name for the solar plexus chakra is Manipura, which means "lustrous gem." Located in the mid-torso, around the navel, this energy center is also found at the middle back. In many ways, the solar plexus serves as our personal energy center, as it relates to our personal identity and power. It is the core of who we are as individuals and governs our self-esteem, willpower, and ability to achieve our goals.

When the solar plexus energies are balanced and flowing, we have a strong sense of self that can't be shaken. This manifests as confidence in who we are and what we want, as well as the belief and grit to accomplish our dreams. The innate self-confidence and ability to be true to ourselves also enable us to transform with the tides of life.

CORRESPONDENCES

COLOR	ELEMENT	SYMBOL	SHAPE
Yellow	Fire		Globe

PLANET (AND STAR)

Mars   The Sun

ASTROLOGICAL SIGNS

Leo   Aries

STONES

Pyrite   Yellow agate
Citrine   Amber

GODDESS ARCHETYPE

The Warrior

ANIMAL

Lion

ESSENTIAL OILS

Lemon   Ginger
Grapefruit   Peppermint

SOLAR PLEXUS CHAKRA IMBALANCE

Since the solar plexus governs the very essence of who we are, if it is not functioning healthily, our lives will be off-kilter. Signs of an overactive solar plexus include being egotistical, controlling, and power hungry. In our quest to get what we want, we may be obsessive and perfectionistic, leading to both disappointment and feeling drained when our desires do not manifest. Too much energy flowing from this chakra can result in being hyperactive and exuding manic energy, then crashing afterward (similar to how you might feel after consuming an energy drink!).

In the case of an underactive solar plexus, we may struggle with being authentic, having self-doubt, and being confused about our identity. This all leads to low self-esteem and insecurity. We may have difficulty manifesting our desires and feel depressed as a result. We may think we are at the mercy of fate and feel that life is happening to, rather than being lived by, us.

The solar plexus rules the parts of the body nearest to it: the abdominal organs, stomach, liver, gallbladder, spleen, and pancreas. When the third chakra is imbalanced, we may experience physical and emotional symptoms such as the following:

- Bloating
- Digestive issues (irritable bowel syndrome, constipation, leaky gut)

- Nausea

- Indigestion

- Fatigue/lethargy

- Difficulty concentrating

- Restlessness

- Agitation

- Gallstones

- Liver issues

- Pancreatic disorders, such as diabetes

WHEN THE SOLAR PLEXUS CHAKRA OPENS

When the solar plexus is activated, we will experience a range of physical and emotional changes along with sensations of heat and tingling vibrations in the area. Given the chakra's proximity to the stomach, we are likely to experience some digestive issues, such as nausea, bloating, constipation, or diarrhea, before it heals.

On an emotional level, it is normal to feel more sensitive than usual. Old insecurities and self-doubts can resurface. We may be easily triggered and feel jealousy and the need for control—the result of a rampant ego rearing its head. It's normal to feel anxiety and emotional disturbances during the opening and rebalancing of the solar plexus, but as with the physical symptoms, this is usually a short-lived purging process. In addition, we may experience fluctuations in our energy as the solar plexus aligns, going from energy highs to lows. We may feel restless, which can result in difficulty sleeping, but rest assured, any insomnia is also usually temporary.

GODDESS ARCHETYPE: THE WARRIOR

The Warrior is a sacred mixture of masculine and feminine energies. This goddess archetype for the solar plexus chakra has a strong sense of self, is spirited and energetic, and has the will and power to pursue her goals. She represents physical strength and energy, leadership, and courage.

There are many historical Warriors revered in different religions and cultures, as well as in art and literature, including Freya, the Norse goddess of love and war; Durga, the multi-limbed Hindu goddess and protector; and Boudicca, the queen of the British Celtic tribe who led the uprising against the Romans. Their names, culture, and race may differ, but they share a very strong sense of self. They were brave and strong and had the willpower and stamina to pursue their causes.

"To thine own self be true," Shakespeare said, and the Warrior goddess reminds us of this. When we consider the essential role the solar plexus chakra plays in both being our true selves and having the belief and resolve to live our best lives, the benefits of taking on the traits of the Warrior are clear. She reminds us that being who we truly are is not only safe but also essential for our well-being. When we become a Warrior, we connect to our power source, we stand up for ourselves and others, and we become strong forces for good in the world, benefiting both our own lives and the world at large.

SOLAR PLEXUS CHAKRA STONES

You will notice that many of the crystals and precious metals that relate to the third chakra have yellow tones, conjuring the sunshine like a life force for this powerful energy point.

PYRITE

Historically confused with gold, pyrite is often referred to as "fool's gold." Pyrite ranges in color from a pale yellow to a vibrant gold or silver. This stone was used in ancient times to create a spark and fire. Thus, we can use pyrite to ignite the spark of our true selves. It has a masculine energy and is a stone of action, strength, and will. As with most stones, you can get raw or polished pyrite. I recommend a fairly large raw pyrite for your desk or workspace and a few smaller tumbled pyrite stones for meditation and rituals.

CITRINE

A beautiful, bright stone with yellowy hues, citrine enhances energy and stamina and represents abundance and manifestation of all sorts. This stone is powered by the sun and can promote confidence and boost self-esteem. A polished citrine point can sit on your altar or desk and is ideally placed in a sunlit space to be charged and then used in meditation or ritual.

YELLOW AGATE

Often known as the revitalizer, yellow agate helps foster self-acceptance, boost self-esteem, and promote positivity. Using a few small tumbled yellow agate stones directly on the solar plexus chakra in healing sessions or meditating with them can foster a ritual of reconnecting to your true self, giving you a regular boost.

AMBER

This bright and cheerful stone helps clear the mind and eliminate fears, all helping align the precious energies of the solar plexus. Wearing jewelry with amber stones can keep the third chakra aligned. Wearing a combination of amber and gold is particularly powerful and one of my favorite ways to connect to my solar plexus.

SOLAR PLEXUS CHAKRA ESSENTIAL OILS

Each of the recommended essential oils for the solar plexus has a refreshing and vibrant scent and vibrant energies to promote the healthy functioning of this energy center.

LEMON

This uplifting and invigorating citrus oil has a powerful energetic influence on the third chakra. Diffusing this oil can bring a sense of well-being and optimism. You can also mix it with a carrier oil and use it as a body moisturizer or massage oil.

GRAPEFRUIT

Grapefruit is another citrus oil that can help move stagnant energy in an underactive solar plexus chakra. This oil's properties help heal digestive issues, so it makes for a powerful massage oil when blended with a carrier. When diffused, its light and fragrant scent can also help reduce stress and lift your spirits.

GINGER

Ginger oil has a very distinct, warm, and spicy aroma and is wonderful for steam inhalation to help awaken the solar plexus chakra. It is also used topically with a carrier oil to stimulate the third chakra and help alleviate any digestive issues.

PEPPERMINT

Peppermint is an invigorating oil that helps to stimulate the mind. Simply sniffing this oil can help provide relief from stress and mental exhaustion. Mixing it with a carrier and dabbing some on your wrists and temples is a helpful way to boost your energy levels and spirits on a daily basis.

PERSONAL POWER BLEND

The purpose of this solar plexus chakra oil blend is to help connect with yourself and empower you to fulfill your true desires. You can use this oil regularly when going through the process of opening and rebalancing your solar plexus, and whenever you need an energetic lift and reminder of your true, powerful essence.

INGREDIENTS

2 tbsp   almond oil (or another carrier oil)
3 drops   lemon essential oil
3 drops   grapefruit essential oil
2 drops   peppermint essential oil

TOOLS/EQUIPMENT

2 oz. dark glass bottle
Dropper

YIELD

Makes 1.5 oz.

1. Pour the almond oil into a dark glass bottle.

2. Using a dropper, add each essential oil. Cover the bottle and swirl lightly.

3. Massage the oil as needed onto your abdomen, mid-back, your temples, and wrists. (For external use only.)

☸ SOLAR PLEXUS CHAKRA VISUALIZATION

As fire is the ruling element of the solar plexus, it is important to have that element present during your visualization meditation exercise. If you have an actual fireplace (whether real or artificial) or fire pit, you may wish to carry out this visualization exercise near it. You'll also draw in the element of fire as you burn sage to cleanse your sacred space and then light a candle. Diffusing lemon oil will help to energetically tap into the solar plexus.

1. Lie down and close your eyes.
2. Take a deep breath in through your nose, exhale out through your mouth, and sigh. Let your muscles soften and your body relax. Repeat this as many times as needed until you feel relaxed and ready for meditation.
3. As you continue to inhale and exhale deeply, visualize your breath as coming in and out of your navel.
4. Keeping your eyes closed, repeat to yourself (either silently or aloud), "I acknowledge and honor my true self, and so I see my solar plexus clearly."
5. Using your mind's eye, visualize a yellow globe at your navel. Look at the exact shade, and notice the size of this globe. Observe its shape. Take note of any other details, including if it is spinning or static. Notice how this globe

feels and what insights you receive about any imbalances or blockages and what you may need to do in order to bring your solar plexus to energetic equilibrium.

6. Once you feel you have observed the globe and obtained sufficient insight into the functioning of your solar plexus chakra, take a moment to acknowledge and give gratitude to this energy point in your body, and then gently open your eyes.

SOLAR PLEXUS CHAKRA ACTIVATION

It is important to bring in the element of fire in order to facilitate the activation of the solar plexus. You will also need to make sure you have warm hands, as you will need the energy from heat to assist with this activation exercise. Light a scented candle (orange, lemon, or grapefruit), as this will be better for activation.

1. You will begin in a standing position, but if you need to, you can sit on a chair or lie down.
2. Look at the flame of the candle you have lit and carefully cup your hands around the flame of the candle to gently heat them.

3. Settle into the position you will stay in for the duration of the activation meditation. Close your eyes, keeping the flame of the candle in your mind's eye.

4. Place your hands over your navel and midsection and breathe into your hands, visualizing the flame of the candle. Envision that yellow light as streaming from your hands and entering your navel with every breath. See this yellow light as pouring from your navel into your belly, where it spins almost like a spool.

5. Bring your mind's eye once again to the yellow globe, which represents your solar plexus chakra. See the yellow light in your belly as filling up this globe. As the globe continues to fill with this yellow light, see it get bigger and brighter until it almost starts to come alive. See the globe beginning to spin in a clockwise direction, picking up speed until it moves so quickly that it's now a whirling spool of bright yellow light that fills your entire midsection.

6. As this light permeates your body, feel the energy of confidence and power flood your being. With every breath, feel that sense of purpose, power, and strength emanating from your navel and spreading across your midsection and entire body. With every breath, feel proud of who you are and confident in your capabilities. Let every breath fuel your fire!

SOLAR PLEXUS CHAKRA REFLECTION

Prepare some hot ginger tea with a slice of lemon. Get settled in your sacred space or another space that feels comfortable to you. Diffuse one or a combination of the solar plexus chakra oils, and light a candle. Gently massage a few drops of your Personal Power Blend (p. 71) around your belly button in a clockwise direction. Have some of the solar plexus chakra stones nearby or hold some in one hand. Place one hand on your navel, and inhale and exhale deeply with your eyes closed. Take as many deep breaths as needed.

Open your eyes, and journal about your experiences of your Solar Plexus Chakra Visualization and Activation. Reflect on what you have learned about your solar plexus chakra and how an imbalanced and/or blocked solar plexus chakra may make you feel. Note whether you are experiencing some of the symptoms or issues discussed and any insights you receive as to what you may need to do for this chakra to be fully open, balanced, and performing optimally. Use the following questions to guide your reflection:

- Do you honor who you are, particularly with friends and family?

- Do you value yourself?

- Are you confident in your abilities to achieve your desires and live the life of your dreams?

- Do you honor your own power and use it appropriately?
- Do you exercise your personal choice and know that you are always free to choose in all situations?
- Do you respect yourself and make choices that reflect that self-respect?
- Are you comfortable with the concept of personal power and with using it when necessary?

❀ SOLAR PLEXUS CHAKRA AFFIRMATIONS

As the solar plexus affirmations are aimed at helping you connect to yourself and be confident in your personal power, they are best done facing a mirror and staring into your own eyes. You can repeat this daily, ideally first thing in the morning. When you are going through the process of opening your solar plexus and balancing it, you can repeat these affirmations as needed. As with all the mantras, you can also repeat them silently and as part of a meditation practice, although for maximum benefit, they are best said aloud.

Gently massage some of your Personal Power Blend (p. 71) or a few drops of lemon or grapefruit oil on your neck, wrists, and temples and around your navel. Stand tall with your feet planted firmly on the ground and your head up high. As you repeat each affirmation, visualize a small flame flickering around your navel and getting stronger and bigger with each affirmation. Feel this flame as the essence of you, your true self, your energy and confidence, growing stronger with the words of each affirmation.

- I know who I am, and I honor and embrace my true self.
- I am confident and open with others as to who I am.
- I am confident in who I am and my ability to create what I desire.
- I believe I am worthy of my desires.
- I have the strength and energy to pursue my passions.
- I am proud of myself and all I have achieved.
- I am comfortable with my personal power and use it wisely.

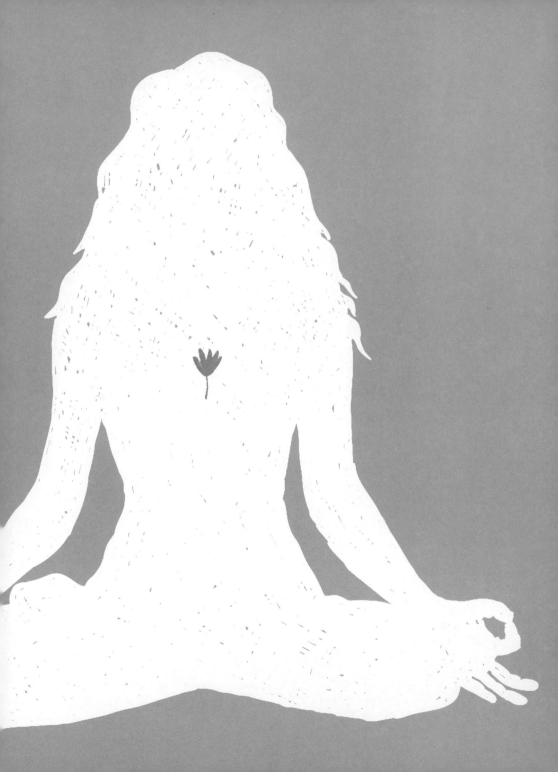

FIVE

HEART CHAKRA

ONE LOVE,
ONE HEART,
ONE DESTINY.

Bob Marley

As the fourth of the main energy centers, the heart chakra is found at the center of the chest and between the shoulder blades in the back. The Sanskrit name for the heart chakra is Anahata, which means "unstruck, unhurt, unbeaten" and gives a nod to the pure loving nature of the fourth chakra.

In many ways, the heart chakra serves as the energy center for love and our ability to both give and receive it, as well as the qualities of compassion, empathy, and forgiveness. It is also the center for connection and facilitates our ability to be connected to all beings and objects. We are able to see the connection between ourselves and the rest of life on Earth. The fourth energy center is considered the energetic bridge between the physical and spiritual realms, acting as a unifier between the three lower chakras, which relate to our human individuality, and the three upper chakras, which are of the spiritual senses and are the realms of our soul.

When the heart chakra is open and flowing well, you will emit a loving energy and be capable of loving yourself and others, and you will receive the love you give. You will feel deeply connected and enjoy harmonious exchanges with others. You will see good in everything and everyone and appreciate beauty in the smallest of details. In that sense, as the ancient sages would say, you will have that spark of the divine. This energy center helps us to realize the interconnectedness that makes us one in contrast to the polarity of much of the other aspects of our lives.

HEART CHAKRA IMBALANCE

As with all the chakras, an imbalance in the heart chakra may mean it is overactive or underactive. In the case of an underactive heart chakra, the energy flow is blocked or stagnant, and we may find our hearts are almost closed off, that we are emotionally closed or numb. We may struggle with giving or receiving love, or we may find it difficult to forgive others or get over past pains. We may be self-isolating, lack empathy or compassion, and feel disconnected from others. We may grapple with self-love and be unduly critical of ourselves and others.

With an overactive heart chakra, there may be too much energy flowing, which means we overly connect to others, leading to

CORRESPONDENCES

COLOR	ELEMENT	SYMBOL	SHAPE
Green	Air		Crescent moon

PLANET

Venus

ASTROLOGICAL SIGNS

Libra   Taurus

STONES

Rose quartz   Emerald

Chrysoprase   Morganite

GODDESS ARCHETYPE

The Lover

ANIMAL

Dove

ESSENTIAL OILS

Rose   Jasmine

Neroli   Lavender

misjudgment, giving too much, or codependency in relationships. We may appear loving to others, but the motivation comes from not feeling complete within ourselves. We may neglect our own emotions and fail to love ourselves, lacking boundaries with others and saying yes even when it is detrimental to us. This can lead to all kinds of imbalances within our lives and can have a negative impact on our overall well-being. Other symptoms of an overactive heart chakra may be fear of abandonment, jealousy, possessiveness, and emotional dependence.

The heart chakra rules the organs and body parts found closest to it: the heart, lungs, respiratory system, thymus, and upper back. When the fourth energy center is imbalanced in some way, we can experience a multitude of physical symptoms, such as the following:

- Chest pain and heart disease
- Respiratory issues, including asthma
- Restlessness, including palpitations
- Shortness of breath
- Panic attacks
- Depression
- Insomnia
- Lack of energy
- Immune system deficiencies
- Shoulder and upper back pain

WHEN THE HEART CHAKRA OPENS

Since the heart chakra rules our emotional energy, when it opens, you may experience a surge of emotions, some that may have been buried and others that you may have thought you dealt with. These can make you feel a deep sense of loss. You may need to process emotions, especially any that you swept under the carpet (in the case of a blocked/inactive heart chakra), or you may suddenly have an emotional hangover, drained and overwhelmed by emotions from an overactive heart chakra.

When your heart chakra opens, this wave of emotion is likely to affect your physical body too. You may feel heart or chest pain, shortness of breath, or even palpitations as you allow yourself to feel once more. You may experience insomnia as you navigate this emotional roller coaster, which can deplete your immune system temporarily, making you prone to sickness.

As always, these symptoms will pass, but the emotions will need processing. You must be kind to yourself and give yourself the space and tools to process them, which in turn will help alleviate any physical discomforts.

GODDESS ARCHETYPE: THE LOVER

The Lover epitomizes the heart chakra. Her mode of operating is to love, connect, and live from a heart-centered place. While many people think that the Lover is all about sex, sensuality, and intimacy, the Lover is actually about so much more. She presides over all love: romantic, familial, platonic, and divine. She seeks unity and connection among all beings, mirroring the oneness of the heart chakra.

The Lover seeks to spread love and connection. She infuses every aspect of her life with love and is dedicated, committed, and faithful. Relationships are her main purpose, and she is unafraid of expressing her emotions, seeing this as an essential part of heart-centered living. Sensual and bohemian, she is in love with love and in love with life. The Lover is a shining example of how to live with an open and flowing heart chakra, seeing the beauty in everyone and everything, and experiencing love in all forms and places.

In history, she was known to the Greeks as Aphrodite and to the Romans as Venus. She is revered in film, art, and literature as a seductress of sorts, but her persona extends far beyond sex and intimacy. The Lover, just like Venus, focuses much of her energy on creating a beautiful life, one she can love. An enthusiast of aesthetics, beauty, nature, and art, the Lover takes time to feel beautiful inside and out (a powerful form of self-care) and creates beautiful environments wherever she goes.

Each of us can turn to the Lover as a role model for how to live from our heart chakra. By taking on her loving traits, we can learn to love ourselves and others and live from a truly heart-centered place, where we see beauty and experience uplifting joy in day-to-day life and can enjoy better relationships of all kinds.

HEART CHAKRA STONES

While some of the stones connected to the heart chakra are pink, the color that traditionally is most associated with the heart chakra and love is green.

ROSE QUARTZ

Rose quartz is the most popular and well-known stone for healing the heart chakra by soothing internal pain and transmuting emotional conditioning. It encourages self-love and self-forgiveness and promotes love and beauty of all sorts. Placing this stone by your bedside is good when you are going through a time of emotional processing and healing. Rose quartz can also help draw in romantic love for those who are seeking it. I used to carry a few pieces of polished rose quartz with me for several years when I was doing the work to call in my soul mate.

MORGANITE

One of my favorite stones, morganite, has pinkish hues similar to rose quartz. Another healer of the heart chakra, morganite helps clear emotional pain and opens the heart to receiving and giving love. It's a very popular stone for facilitating shifts with romantic love, and wearing this beautiful heart-lifting stone as jewelry can help heal old wounds and draw in romantic love.

CHRYSOPRASE

A cheerful and uplifting green stone, chrysoprase is wonderful for meditation, as it helps us with personal insights, remembering our divine connection, and facilitating our connection to all beings. This stone is also excellent for healing deep emotional trauma and anxiety and helping us forgive ourselves and others for past events. Holding a polished chrysoprase when meditating or having it on your altar and/or bedside while opening and balancing the heart chakra will help with this process.

EMERALD

Known as the stone of successful love, emerald promotes unity, unconditional love, loyalty, and partnership. This stone helps harmonize relationships of all sorts, but it is particularly powerful for promoting domestic bliss. While emerald has a calming effect on emotions, it also acts as an invigorator for the mind. It's a lovely stone to wear as jewelry, as a beautiful way of facilitating the openness of the heart chakra. Be mindful, however, of overstimulation; wearing or using emerald all the time is unnecessary and not recommended.

HEART CHAKRA ESSENTIAL OILS

Perhaps unsurprisingly, the recommended essential oils for the heart chakra are sweet and feminine, helping us tap into the divine feminine energy of this powerful chakra.

ROSE

Soft and sweet, rose evokes feelings of love, so it is no surprise that it's one of the most powerful scents for working with the heart chakra. Simply sniffing the scent of rose oil can help calm the heart and mind. You can also diffuse it to help permeate your space with loving, calming energy. I personally like to dab a bit of this oil on my chest and neck to really connect to the heart center. It's also a marvelous oil to mix with a carrier oil and use in massage.

JASMINE

Another sweet and sensual essential oil is jasmine, which is known for its aphrodisiacal properties but is also fantastic for calming our emotions and relieving the anger and stress that can be associated with harboring old wounds. Diffusing this oil in any space automatically creates a calming and sensual environment. I highly recommend using this oil in a room or as a personal spray.

LAVENDER

A versatile oil, lavender can be used for all the chakras. It is particularly potent at healing emotional stress that can be felt through the heart chakra and releasing feelings of self-doubt. It is very calming and relaxing and is wonderful mixed with a carrier oil for massage purposes, diffused, or directly inhaled. A dab of lavender oil on the chest and temples can help in heart chakra rituals and meditations.

NEROLI

Neroli oil comes from the blossoms of an orange tree and has a distinctive exotic, citrus, floral scent. Popular as a blend in massage oils, neroli oil has a sensual undertone that helps promote physical connection, but it also has a soothing effect. Diffuse neroli oil or inhale it directly to help open the heart chakra and to encourage trust and promote a sense of security, which will allow love in.

COMPASSION AND CONNECTION BLEND

Use this oil blend when you're going through the process of opening and rebalancing your heart chakra. This blend will help you heal and open your heart center and practice compassion, allowing you to connect to yourself and to others more easily.

INGREDIENTS

2 tbsp jojoba oil (or another carrier oil)
3 drops rose essential oil
2 drops jasmine essential oil
2 drops lavender essential oil
1 drop neroli essential oil

TOOLS/EQUIPMENT

2 oz. dark glass bottle
Dropper

YIELD

Makes 1.5 oz.

1. Pour the jojoba oil (my favorite for the heart chakra) into a dark glass bottle.

2. Using a dropper, add each essential oil. Cover the bottle and swirl lightly.

3. Massage the oil as needed onto your chest, mid-back, temples, or wrists. (For external use only.)

☸ HEART CHAKRA VISUALIZATION

You can prepare for your visualization meditation with a little tender loving self-care. Take a cleansing bath or shower, perhaps using rose- or lavender-scented products. (My personal favorite is to add rose petals to a bath and use rose-scented bath salts.) After your bath, apply the Compassion and Connection Blend (p. 89) or rose oil directly on your chest. You can also add it to your moisturizer and apply it to your entire body. In your sacred space, smudge using a white sage bundle or palo santo to clear the energy. Diffuse one or a combination of the heart chakra essential oils, or light a rose incense stick, and put a heart chakra stone in your hand.

1. Lie down and close your eyes.
2. Take a deep breath in through your nose, exhale through your mouth, and sigh. Let your muscles soften and your body relax. Repeat this as many times as needed until you feel relaxed and ready for meditation.
3. Continuing to inhale and exhale deeply, place one hand on your chest and visualize your breath coming in and out of your heart center.
4. Keeping your eyes closed, repeat to yourself (either silently or aloud), "I know that love is the essence of

who I am and the purpose of my existence, and so I see my heart chakra."

5. Now, visualize a green crescent moon at your chest. Look at the exact shade, and notice the size of this crescent moon. Observe its dimensions and any other noticeable details, including if it is spinning or static. Notice how this crescent moon feels and what insights you receive about any imbalances or blockages, or what you may need to do to bring your heart chakra to energetic equilibrium.

6. Once you feel you have observed the crescent moon and obtained sufficient insight into the functioning of your heart chakra, take a moment to acknowledge and give gratitude to this energy point in your body. Gently open your eyes.

❀ HEART CHAKRA ACTIVATION

Given the nature and function of the heart chakra, it would be sensible to prepare for the activation by indulging in a little self-care. Whether that is enjoying a facial, a body treatment, or a simple, relaxing bubble bath, show yourself some tender loving care to best facilitate the opening and aligning of your heart center. As always, clear your sacred space to set the tone for the smoothest facilitation of this Heart Chakra Activation. Conduct a sage-burning ceremony, and then diffuse a combination of the heart chakra oils to create an ambiance of relaxation and connection. Wearing the color green, especially as a top, can also help activate the heart chakra.

This activation is best performed either lying down or seated. Once you are in a comfortable position, close your eyes and take a few moments to get settled, focusing on breathing slowly and fully, relaxing and loosening the muscles in your body, so you feel soft and supple.

1. Place one hand over your heart center and one over your belly. Begin to breathe into your belly, sending that breath up into your heart center and feeling it expand and rise. As you exhale, feel your chest drop as the air leaves your body, contracting your belly.

2. Repeat this a few times with slow, deep breaths, and start to visualize a green light filling your chest with your breath as you inhale and exhale.

3. Bring your mind's eye to the green crescent moon at your chest, which represents your heart chakra. See the green light fill up this crescent moon, which starts to grow in size and vividness with each breath. See the moon growing so large that it fills your entire chest area and then slowly begins to spin, picking up speed until you can no longer see the moon and it is simply a

vibrant whirling green light that floods your chest and
the rest of your body.

4. As this green light infuses your body, bring both hands to
   your chest and feel your chest expand and soften. Visualize
   the energy flowing from this green moon and your heart
   chakra throughout your body. You can visualize this as a
   green light that permeates your entire physical being.

5. As you see and feel this energy flooding your body, feel
   love and compassion for yourself, and feel that sense of
   love fill your entire physical being with joy. Gently open
   your eyes when you are finished.

✿ HEART CHAKRA REFLECTION

Prepare some chamomile, rose, or lavender tea (a combination of rose
and chamomile is delicious). Next, diffuse some heart chakra essential
oils, or light a rose- or jasmine-scented candle or incense stick. Collect
your heart chakra crystals, and take a few minutes to hold them in one
hand while sipping your tea, connecting to the power of these precious
stones. Take a few drops of your Compassion and Connection Blend
(p. 89) or jasmine oil and dab it onto your neck, wrists, and temples.
Gently massage a drop or two onto your chest. Take a few deep breaths
in and out of your heart center with your eyes closed.

Gently open your eyes and jot down your experience of your Heart Chakra Visualization and Activation. Reflect on what you have learned about your heart chakra and the underactive or overactive symptoms. Note whether you have felt any of these symptoms or issues, as well as any other insights you may have as to what you need for your heart center to be fully open and flowing healthily. Use these questions to guide you:

- Do you love yourself and others?
- Can you forgive yourself and others?
- Do you love life?
- Do you feel at peace?
- Do you believe that we are all connected?
- Can you see the connection between yourself and others?
- How do you experience joy in your life, and what would you like to do to cultivate more joy?

❀ HEART CHAKRA AFFIRMATIONS

Heart chakra affirmations should be repeated multiple times a day when opening and aligning the heart chakra. Given that self-love is the foundation from which we achieve milestones in our lives, it's useful to repeat these affirmations regularly to remind yourself of your true essence, allowing you to honor yourself and connect better with others. As with all the affirmations, you can also repeat them silently and as part of a meditation practice, although for maximum benefit, they are best repeated out loud for at least part of your ritual.

To begin, gently massage some of your Compassion and Connection Blend (p. 89) or rose oil on your chest. Stand or sit tall with your feet planted firmly on the ground and your head held high. As you repeat each affirmation, visualize a green light entering into your heart center and becoming brighter and more vivid with each affirmation. Feel this light as the pure, loving essence of your true self. With each affirmation, feel a sense of love, peace, and joy flooding your entire heart center and body.

- I know that in truth we are all connected, and love is our true essence.
- I operate from a foundation of love.
- I feel love and compassion for myself and others.
- I am at peace with myself and others.
- I find joy and connection in everyday life.
- I love fully and freely.
- Love is flowing toward me and through me at all times.
- I radiate love, and it is returned to me exponentially.
- The universe surrounds me with love.
- I see and experience beauty everywhere I go.

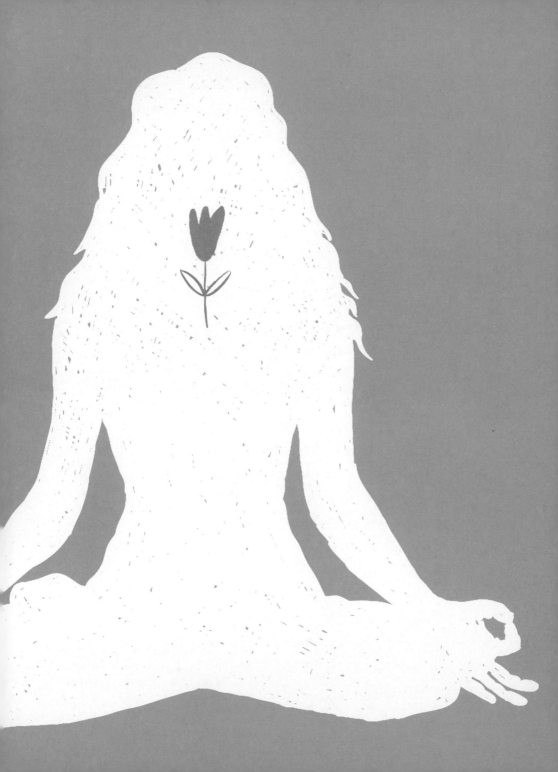

SIX

THROAT CHAKRA

**WORDS HAVE THE POWER
TO BOTH DESTROY AND
HEAL. WHEN WORDS ARE
BOTH TRUE AND KIND, THEY
CAN CHANGE OUR WORLD.**

Buddha

A s the fifth chakra, the throat chakra is also the first of what is known as the upper chakras (comprising the throat, third eye, and crown), which are considered to be the spiritual and meta-physical energy centers. The throat chakra serves as the entrance to the higher spiritual realms. Ancient mystics often referred to this chakra, when healthy, as the "mouth of God," the notion being that we can both hear and speak divine wisdom and give voice to our soul. As its name suggests, it is found in the throat but is associated with the mouth, tongue, neck, ears, and thyroid and parathyroid glands. The Sanskrit name for the throat chakra is Vishuddha, which

CORRESPONDENCES

COLOR	ELEMENT	SYMBOL	SHAPE
Turquoise blue	Ether		Inverted pyramid

PLANET	ASTROLOGICAL SIGNS
Mercury	Gemini Virgo

STONES	GODDESS ARCHETYPE
Lapis lazuli Aquamarine Blue agate Turquoise	The Communicator

ANIMAL	ESSENTIAL OILS
Elephant	Eucalyptus Tea tree Clove Peppermint

loosely translates to "purity." Shuddhi means "pure" in Sanskrit, and vi placed before shuddhi intensifies the word (vi is a root), so it literally means "especially pure."

The throat chakra is the energy center for speech and communication and is directly linked to our integrity and morals. As this energy point also governs the ears, it allows us to hear the inner voice of our intuition. When this energy center is open and balanced, we also have the capacity for creative expression.

THROAT CHAKRA IMBALANCE

An unbalanced throat chakra can result in a plethora of physical, emotional, and spiritual issues, depending on whether the chakra is over- or underperforming. In the case of an overactive throat chakra, you may find yourself being overly critical or judgmental of others and may express this by gossiping. You may talk nonstop and be extremely loud or shrill; you may even shout. Your mode of communication may be domineering, leading to you talk over people and dominate conversations. At the same time, the nonstop chatter and loudness prevents you from hearing your inner voice, and so you live out of sync with your truth. To compensate, you may find yourself overanalyzing and intellectualizing everything to avoid the vulnerability of facing your emotions and understanding your true feelings.

With an underactive throat chakra, you are likely to suppress your feelings and be fearful of speaking your truth. You may be shy and stumble over your words or even stutter. You swallow your words, more often than not at the cost of being authentic and compromising your integrity. This may manifest as introversion, shyness, insecurity, and speaking too softly or timidly. You may also struggle with owning your creativity and feel an artistic block, suppressing your ideas and insights.

Signs of imbalance of the throat chakra can be felt physically and emotionally and can include the following symptoms:

- Speech impediments, including stuttering and lisps
- Sore throat or laryngitis
- Jaw or mouth pain
- Throat infections
- Sores in mouth
- Hearing issues
- Ear infections
- Neck pain
- Thyroid disorders
- Hormonal imbalances

WHEN THE THROAT CHAKRA OPENS

As the throat chakra essentially rules our voice, when it opens, you are likely to find words effortlessly flowing out and you won't be able to help saying what you think. You may suddenly find yourself unable to stop talking or singing, whereas in the past, you found yourself biting your tongue. Sudden creative rushes and a need to communicate and express yourself through any form of your "voice"—singing, speaking, writing, and so on—are surefire signs that your throat chakra is opening. As you go through the process of balancing this chakra, you may find you lose your voice or have throat or neck issues, which temporarily make it hard for you to physically speak.

Since this chakra also rules our inner voice as well as our ears, be prepared to hear your conscience much more loudly. Having a journal nearby can be useful during the process of opening and aligning your throat chakra, because you may have many intuitive and creative ideas. As with the opening of any of the chakras, it is normal to experience some emotional turbulence.

In the case of an underactive throat chakra, as you start to speak your truth and express your real feelings, you may experience the release of suppressed emotions. During my own process of aligning this chakra, I found myself screaming, roaring, and shouting out all the things I had stifled for so many years and then crying so hard I thought I would run out of tears. I didn't run out of tears, but I did stop crying. While this was temporarily emotionally draining, it was also hugely cathartic, and within days, I not only felt better but was also able to hear my intuition much more clearly, and I had many creative insights. It led to the birth of many projects and I couldn't stop journaling! The pain had a purpose.

As you balance an overactive throat chakra, you may feel guilt and shame at prior interactions and may experience emotional pain as you process your feelings. As always, any healing crisis is temporary and is a necessary part of resetting your mind, body, and soul.

GODDESS ARCHETYPE: THE COMMUNICATOR

The Communicator epitomizes the highest octaves of the throat chakra. Clear and concise, she is as good a listener as she is a talker. Speaking her truth comes naturally, and her voice resonates with others as sincere. She knows when to remain silent and when to speak up. She is creative and expressive and is an uplifting role model to others, helping them connect to their own divine truth. She lives with integrity and is both open-minded and discerning, and she is informed and is an informer. The Communicator displays emotions as opposed to suppressing them, knowing that there is a way to process emotions through healthy expression.

Across history, and in mythology, art, and literature, the Communicator archetype has usually been attributed to a male figure, such as Hermes in Greek mythology or Mercury in Roman mythology. As with each of the archetypes, the Communicator can be male or female, so for our purposes, think of a role model (whether from the past or the present, a real person or a fictitious character) who embodies the traits described above. By adopting the qualities of the Communicator, we can learn to speak our truth, express ourselves, speak up when needed, stay silent when appropriate, and use our voices as a force for good.

THROAT CHAKRA STONES

You will notice that many of the stones connected to the throat chakra are blue and similar to the governing color of the throat chakra, making them potent for activating and balancing this energy center.

AQUAMARINE

This sea-blue stone has extremely calming energies and facilitates the kind of soothing energy we receive when we spend time in or near the ocean. Aquamarine is one of the most powerful stones for opening the throat chakra and bringing it into alignment. I like to mediate lying down with a small polished aquamarine stone gently placed by my throat to help me speak with clarity and confidence.

TURQUOISE

Noted for its protective qualities, turquoise is a healing stone that promotes spiritual connection and, in many ways, paves the path for the soul to express itself once more. When going through the process of opening and aligning the throat chakra, it is very helpful to wear a piece of jewelry with turquoise, ideally a necklace, as this will be near the throat.

BLUE LACE AGATE

This beautiful stone is another powerful healer and balancer of the throat chakra. It alleviates some of the physical symptoms associated with a stagnant fifth chakra due to stifling our thoughts and feelings. Blue lace agate also facilitates the expression of spiritual and personal truths. I like to have a piece of raw blue lace agate on my desk in my sacred space where I journal, as it helps me to connect to my inner truth and express it fully in words.

LAPIS LAZULI

Favored in ancient Egypt as a royal stone said to contain the soul of the gods, lapis lazuli emphasizes the power of the spoken word and brings harmony between our mind, emotions, body, and spirit. It is an exceptionally high vibrational stone, which stimulates our higher mind and promotes creativity. A medium-sized, polished lapis lazuli globe is a wonderful meditation aid that you can hold or place nearby.

THROAT CHAKRA ESSENTIAL OILS

All of the recommended throat chakra essential oils have a very potent scent and decongesting qualities, both of which clear the physical parts of the body ruled by this chakra, helping this energy center to operate fully.

EUCALYPTUS

Refreshing and stimulating to the mind, eucalyptus oil has a bright, clean, and uplifting scent. It supports a clear airway, and energetically it promotes a clear mind and communication. During the process of aligning and opening the throat chakra, you can use eucalyptus, directly sniffed or infused, to alleviate physical symptoms of imbalance, such as a stuffy nose and/or sore throat.

CLOVE

Native to Southeast Asia and true to its roots, clove oil has a rather strong and spicy aroma. It has antimicrobial and pain-relieving qualities and is often used to treat respiratory conditions. Clove oil is useful for opening the throat chakra and dealing with physical imbalance symptoms. Gargling with a few drops of clove oil in warm water a couple times a day is a good ritual for the fifth chakra.

TEA TREE

Also known as melaleuca oil, tea tree has a distinctive medicinal aroma, and this cleansing oil is used for all kinds of medicinal purposes, such as treating colds, wounds, infections, sore throats, and skin conditions (my favorite for pimples!). This is a wonderful oil to use in a simple DIY spray to cleanse your sacred space and yourself when you are working on opening the throat chakra.

PEPPERMINT

Peppermint oil has a fresh, minty, and uplifting aroma and contains menthol, which induces a cooling sensation. I like to add a few drops of peppermint oil to a steam inhalation to help clear my head and sinuses whenever I need an energetic shift before a creative brainstorming session or important interaction.

CLEAR COMMUNICATION BLEND

The purpose of this throat chakra oil blend is to help you express yourself with authenticity, clarity, and confidence. It will aid the process of opening the fifth chakra, balancing it and keeping it in harmonious alignment. You can use it regularly during the alignment of the throat chakra and as needed at other times.

INGREDIENTS

2 tbsp   coconut oil (or another carrier oil)
2 drops eucalyptus essential oil
2 drops peppermint essential oil
1 drop   clove essential oil
1 drop   tea tree essential oil

TOOLS/EQUIPMENT

2 oz. dark glass bottle
Dropper

YIELD

Makes 1.5 oz.

1. Pour the coconut oil into a dark glass bottle.

2. Using a dropper, add each essential oil. Cover the bottle and swirl lightly.

3. Massage the oil onto your neck and throat area and inhale directly as needed. (For external use only.)

☸ THROAT CHAKRA VISUALIZATION

It is important to clear your head and respiratory system before the visualization meditation. Perform a steam inhalation with a mixture of peppermint and tea tree oils. Smudge your sacred space using a white sage bundle or palo santo, and then diffuse some eucalyptus oil. Take a few drops of your Clear Communication Blend (p. 106) or peppermint oil and gently massage it into your neck and throat area. Gather some of your throat chakra stones so they can energetically assist you.

1. Lie down and close your eyes.
2. Take a deep breath in through your nose, exhale through your mouth, and sigh. Let your muscles soften and your body relax. Repeat this as many times as needed until you feel relaxed and ready for meditation.
3. Continue to inhale and exhale deeply, and gently cup your hands around your neck, visualizing your breath entering in and out of your hands.
4. Keeping your eyes closed, repeat to yourself out loud, "I know the value of clear and authentic communication and the power of my words. With this in mind, I honor the energetic center of my voice and creative expression and see it clearly now."

5. Visualize a blue inverted pyramid at your throat, under your hands. (You can also remove your hands if you are uncomfortable and simply focus your mind's eye on your throat). Look closely at this pyramid, noticing its exact shade of blue, its size, and any other details. Observe its dimensions and whether it is spinning or static. Note how this pyramid feels and what insights you received about any imbalances or blockages your throat chakra may have and what you may need to do in order to bring it into a harmonious balance.
6. Once you feel you have observed the pyramid and obtained sufficient insight into the functioning of your throat chakra, take a moment to acknowledge and give gratitude to this energy point in your body, and then gently open your eyes.

THROAT CHAKRA ACTIVATION

Take some time to purify both yourself and your space to best facilitate the powerful divine activation of this fifth chakra. (A suggested pre-activation ritual is a cleansing shower or bath with a few drops of eucalyptus oil.) Cleanse your space by smudging using white sage or Palo Santo. Pour a couple drops of your Clear Communication

Blend (p. 106) or eucalyptus oil onto your throat chakra stones and have them close by, as you will be using them in your activation.

1.   This activation is best performed lying down or seated. Once in a comfortable position, close your eyes and take a few moments to get settled, focusing on breathing slowly and fully, relaxing and loosening the muscles in your body, so you feel soft and supple.

2.   Take one of your polished throat chakra stones moistened with oil and gently rub it across your neck, focusing your attention on the throat area. If comfortable, you can leave the stone there at the base of your neck.

3.   Begin to visualize your breath as a beautiful blue light entering into your throat as you inhale and flooding your entire neck as you exhale.

4.   Bring your mind's eye to a blue inverted pyramid, which represents your throat chakra. Visualize this at the base of your throat. See your breath and that vivid blue light filling up the blue pyramid, making it solid. With each inhalation and exhalation, see the blue pyramid getting bigger and brighter until it fills your entire neck.

5.   Visualize the blue light flowing from this pyramid into the rest of your body, and feel any blocks or barriers to your truthful expression dissipate. Allow yourself to feel

a sense of confidence and peace as you are able to hear your inner voice, tap into your intuition, and receive divine expression. Feel inspired to both speak up and communicate your truth as you see that blue light swirling around your body.

6. With every breath, feel a sense of confidence and peace that you can listen, speak, and create for your highest good and the greater good of all. Allow yourself to make some noise using your voice. Perhaps you could hum, repeat a mantra, sing, or shout.

7. Visualize the energy flowing from this blue pyramid and your throat chakra throughout your body. You can visualize this as a turquoise light that permeates your entire physical being.

8. As you sense this energy flooding your body, feel a deep sense of gratitude for the healthy functioning of this energy center. Gently open your eyes when you are finished.

❁ THROAT CHAKRA REFLECTION

First, prepare some refreshing mint tea. Gather your throat chakra stones and place them near where you will be writing in your journal. Diffuse some eucalyptus and tea tree oils. Gently massage a few drops of your Clear Communication Blend (p. 106) or another throat chakra essential oil onto your neck and throat area. Dab a few drops onto your temples and wrists, and take a few deep inhalations of the blend.

Now turn to your journal, and jot down any reflections you may have on the Throat Chakra Visualization and Activation. Consider what you have learned about your throat chakra, particularly about the imbalances. Reflect on whether you have felt any of these symptoms or issues, and reflect on any intuitive insights regarding the energies of the throat chakra and what you need to do to ensure you are expressing yourself and communicating fully and authentically. Use these questions to guide your reflection:

- Are you open, honest, and clear in all of your communication?
- Do you know when to speak and when to remain silent?
- Are you honest with yourself and with others?
- Do you tune in to your mind, body, and soul to know what your truth is?
- Can you see the connection between creativity and your unique spirit?
- How can you be more creative in your life?
- Do you allow yourself to express yourself creatively in some form?

☙ THROAT CHAKRA AFFIRMATIONS

Throat chakra affirmations should be repeated multiple times a day when going through the opening and aligning process. These affirmations are also helpful for an energetic boost before an important conversation, to communicate openly, or for creative endeavors. These affirmations are best spoken, sung, or shouted, so you feel your voice as you affirm your divine right to communicate and express yourself openly and authentically.

To help with this process, breathe in one of the throat chakra essential oils by sniffing it or using a steam inhalation. Dab some of the Clear Communication Blend (p. 106) or peppermint oil on your neck. Stand or sit tall, drop your shoulders, lift your head high, and straighten your neck. As you repeat each mantra, visualize a bright blue light entering your neck and coming out of your mouth. Allow this light to infuse you with confidence and clarity, as you honor and express your truth.

- I know it is safe and it is my divine right for me to speak my truth.
- I embrace my voice and I speak up.
- I communicate with clarity and confidence.
- I know the power of both my words and silence.
- I know when to listen to others and when to speak.

- I am honest about who I am and what I feel.

- I enjoy expressing myself and finding creative ways to do so.

- I live in my truth. I speak my truth. I am my truth.

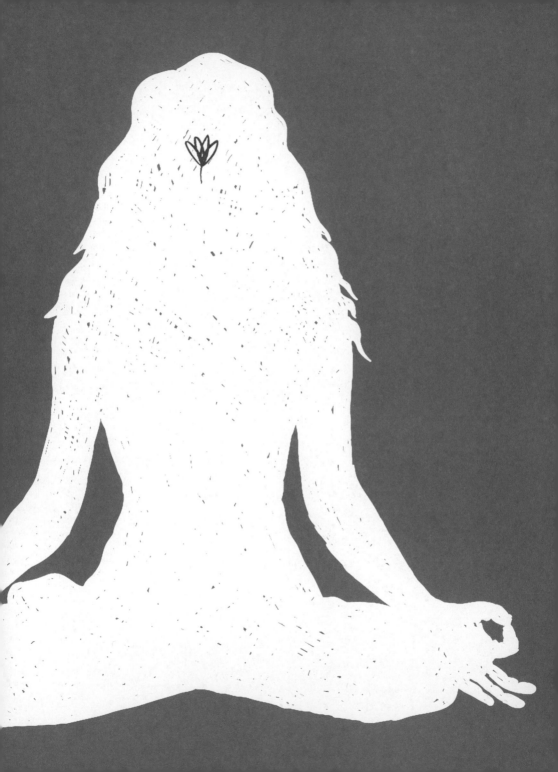

SEVEN

BROW CHAKRA

INTUITION IS SEEING WITH
THE SOUL.

Dean Koontz

The brow chakra is the sixth primary energy point in the body and is found on the forehead between the eyebrows. The sixth chakra is also often referred to as the third eye, or pineal chakra, which gives a nod to its Sanskrit name of Ajna, which translates to "perceive" and "beyond wisdom."

The brow chakra is the energy center for our mind. Ancient sages considered this chakra to be the seat of psychic ability, as it governs our intuition and foresight. It is known as the third eye because it is an invisible eye that "sees" things that aren't necessarily visible. When it is fully activated and flowing harmoniously, this chakra stimulates both the right (creative and spiritual) and left (logical and rational) hemispheres of the brain to work together so the mind can function from a grounded place. A fully functioning brow chakra allows us to trust our intuition, be comfortable in our chosen path, and be able to use both our feelings and facts to make big decisions; as a result, we feel as though we are living in harmony within ourselves.

BROW CHAKRA IMBALANCE

In the case of an overactive brow chakra, we may feel intense psychological and physical symptoms. On a mental level, we are likely to feel overwhelmed and exhausted. Our imagination may be in overdrive, therefore clouding our intuition and our ability to discern between facts and feelings. We may be overly subjective, viewing everything through a limited lens, resulting in our being narrow-minded and inflexible. We may over-intellectualize at the expense of our emotional or spiritual needs. We may have a distorted self-image and struggle with self-acceptance, which includes acceptance of our shadow side. This is essentially our unconscious self—the characteristics and almost automatic behaviors that are deeply rooted within our subconscious and often manifest as negative traits or behaviors. We each have a shadow side, and the point is not to eliminate it but rather to understand it and work to transform it. In some cases of an overactive brow chakra, we may find our clairvoyant skills are overactive, becoming overwhelming and even a bit frightening. (This happened to me, and it was intense and disorienting!)

CORRESPONDENCES

COLOR	ELEMENT	SYMBOL	SHAPE
Indigo	Light		☆ Five-pointed star

PLANETS

4   ♄

Jupiter   Saturn

ASTROLOGICAL SIGNS

Sagittarius   Capricorn

STONES

Sapphire   Labradorite

Celestite   Azurite

GODDESS ARCHETYPE

The Wise Woman

ANIMAL

Hawk

ESSENTIAL OILS

Sandalwood   Patchouli

Bergamot   Vetiver

With an underactive or blocked brow chakra, we are likely to lack a sense of purpose and belief in our chosen path. We may feel energetically drained and uninspired and struggle to find a deeper meaning in our lives. This makes us feel disheartened, skeptical, and fearful of the unknown. When the third eye is blocked, we are unable to either see or connect to our intuition or we mistrust any intuitive notions. We may think we never dream, whereas in truth, we do, but as we are not connected to our subconscious, we are prevented from remembering our dreams and receiving their guidance and wisdom. As this sixth chakra is such an important source of energy for our minds, in the event of blockages, we are likely to struggle with concentration, have difficulty processing information, and be very indecisive.

The sixth energy center governs the pituitary and pineal glands, our neurological system, and our eyes, ears, and nose. Common physical ailments of a blocked brow chakra include the following:

- Migraines
- Sinus issues
- Blurred vision
- Eye strain
- Cataracts
- Glaucoma
- Hallucinations
- Insomnia

- Immune system deficiencies
- High blood pressure
- Hormonal imbalances
- Compromised adrenal function (adrenal fatigue)

WHEN THE BROW CHAKRA OPENS

When the brow chakra opens, you may feel a sense of pressure in between your brows, almost as though that invisible third eye is opening up. When my brow chakra was opened by a healer, I felt an actual pop and saw with my mind's eye a burst of violet light in between my brows. It was an extraordinary experience.

Your third eye opening may not be as dramatic, but as with all the chakras, you may experience a sense of tingling and warmth as energy begins to flow. This may make your physical eyes more sensitive to light. Some people experience a temporary blurriness in vision or a noticeable increase in the vividness of colors; this may be subtle or more obvious, depending on your unique journey. Headaches are another symptom of the brow chakra opening and a sign that the pineal gland is regulating itself. As this gland produces and regulates many hormones, including melatonin, which impacts our ability to sleep, it is possible to experience some disruption to sleeping habits. Whether this means you suddenly can't get enough sleep and are sleeping in way past your alarm or you experience insomnia and restlessness, remember that as with all the chakra opening systems, this is temporary. As the saying goes, this too shall pass.

As the third eye opens and balances, so too will your intuitive ability awaken, so you may suddenly be flooded with insights and an increase in foresight. Keeping a notebook handy is useful for this time so you can jot down your thoughts. A somewhat disruptive result of the third eye opening is an increase in clairvoyance, which can be overwhelming or even a little frightening. Rest assured, this is part of rebalancing, and you can bring your clairvoyant ability to a healthy flow that helps you and others, rather than frightening or hindering you.

GODDESS ARCHETYPE: THE WISE WOMAN

The Wise Woman is, as her name suggests, a wise soul. She is revered by others for her wisdom and knowledge. Both practical and spiritual, she is the voice of reason but also a voice of inspiration and faith in what is unseen yet felt. The Wise Woman is the result of a fully balanced brow chakra, as she operates with balance between facts and feelings, logic and intuition, reality and alternative paradigms. She is knowledgeable in facts and has insights that come from higher sources: her intuition, her higher self, and her divine connection to God and the universe.

Kind, compassionate, and wise, she is also mysterious, magical, and prophetic. She is a heroine to herself and many others and is seen as a protector, not dissimilar to the Mother archetype, but in a less nurturing and more detached way, yet she is still compassionate. In history and folklore and literature, the Wise Woman is more often than not portrayed as an older woman—but the truth is that the Wise Woman is seen for her wisdom, not her age. The young wise person you think of as an "old soul" is an example of the Wise Woman. She is the fairy godmother or queen in fairy tales, or the wise mysterious figure in literature, the one who "sees it all" and speaks from her mind and soul, and whose wisdom and guidance are sought by others.

The Wise Woman teaches us that we, too, can be a balance of our minds, hearts, and souls, and can operate from a place of deep inner wisdom. We can adopt her traits to be logical and objective, yet also allow our intuition to divinely guide us. By paying attention to small details and facts and trusting in the bigger picture and our feelings, we can pursue our purpose with a sense of confidence and alignment, and we can pursue our dreams and live our lives with faith in both the seen and the unseen.

BROW CHAKRA STONES

All of the brow chakra stones are highly vibrational and have powerful mystical qualities associated with this energy center.

SAPPHIRE

Given that Saturn is one of the planets that governs the brow chakra, this beautiful indigo gem gets its name from the Sanskrit word sanipriya, which means "dear to the planet Saturn." Sapphire is regarded as the wisdom stone, as it helps calm and focus the mind, releasing unnecessary mental chatter and tension. Placing a polished sapphire stone in between your brows is a wonderful way to help clear the brow chakra and bring it into alignment.

CELESTITE

One of the highest vibrational stones I have come across, celestite stimulates spiritual development and promotes trust in divine energy. This stone is one of my favorites for balancing the brow chakra, as it not only calms emotions but also integrates our intellect and logical mind with our feelings and intuitive mind, bringing equilibrium between both sides of the brain. I like to have a piece of raw celestite on my altar, and I use celestite wands or small polished stones in meditation.

LABRADORITE

The stone of transformation, labradorite is a highly mystical and protective stone that helps raise your consciousness by removing fears and insecurities and other emotional baggage that clouds your mind and diminishes your ability to think clearly and hear your intuition. Labradorite is a powerful stone to use when opening and activating the brow chakra. You can use a collection of small polished labradorite stones or one medium-sized stone directly on your brow chakra.

AZURITE

Known as the psychic's stone, azurite ranges from dark blue to indigo, and its vibrational energy matches that of the brow chakra. A wonderful stone to awaken our intuition and psychic abilities, as well as open our minds to spiritual and divine wisdom, it is an important stone for both activating and balancing the third eye and is useful in ritual and meditation. Raw azurite is simply stunning and my preferred form of this stone.

BROW CHAKRA ESSENTIAL OILS

You may recognize some of the recommended essential oils for the brow chakra, as they are mentioned in earlier chapters for other energy centers. Often, an essential oil will be beneficial for multiple chakras.

SANDALWOOD

This is a go-to essential oil for balancing each of the chakras, as it is highly beneficial for meditation and ritual purposes. It also stimulates the pituitary and pineal glands, thus helping the entire endocrine system, which produces various hormones for the body. Diffusing this oil, inhaling it directly, or using it in an essential oil blend can all help during the opening of the brow chakra and enhance spiritual and intuitive awareness.

BERGAMOT

Citrusy, spicy bergamot oil is highly regarded for aromatherapy. This oil has a distinctive aroma, which both calms and enlivens. It also promotes the release of old, negative, and outdated thought patterns that can imbalance the brow chakra. By dabbing a few drops of diluted bergamot oil directly on the space between your brows, you can open and heal this energy center.

VETIVER

One of my favorite essential oils, vetiver has a beautiful earthy, spicy aroma that is instantly grounding and calming. This oil can be used in a variety of ways to calm and ground an overactive brow chakra, as it soothes anxiety, which then releases negative and fearful thoughts, bringing clarity to the mind. Vetiver also allows you to think clearly and receive intuitive guidance. I enjoy adding a few drops of vetiver oil to a hot bath to help me relax and obtain clarity.

PATCHOULI

Warm, spicy, and sensuous, patchouli is another essential oil that is beneficial for many of the chakras thanks to its balancing and grounding properties. Some of the constituents of patchouli are helpful for lifting spirits and balancing emotions when dealing with a closed or imbalanced brow chakra. As patchouli has some sedative effects, diffusing this oil at night can relieve some sleep-related issues and provide energetic assistance when you are going through the process of aligning this chakra.

CLEAR MIND AND VISION BLEND

The purpose of this oil blend is to help you clear and calm your mind, so you can access your intuition more easily and think and act from your higher self. As with all the chakra blends, this custom blend is helpful when activating and balancing the brow chakra, but it's also beneficial to use at times when you feel uncertain, confused, or fearful and need to connect to your intuition and receive divine guidance.

INGREDIENTS

2 tbsp almond oil (or other carrier oil)
2 drops sandalwood essential oil
2 drops bergamot essential oil
1 drop vetiver essential oil
1 drop patchouli essential oil

TOOLS/EQUIPMENT

2 oz. dark glass bottle
Dropper

YIELD

Makes 1.5 oz.

1. Pour the almond oil into a dark glass bottle.

2. Using a dropper, add each essential oil. Cover the bottle and swirl lightly.

3. Massage or dab the oil onto your forehead, between your brows, and onto your neck as needed. Inhale directly for instant energetic assistance. (For external use only.)

✿ BROW CHAKRA VISUALIZATION

A clear space leads to a clear mind. If you are performing this visualization exercise in your sacred space, it should already be clean and tidy. You should still conduct a smudging exercise, using white sage or palo santo to energetically clear the space and set the tone. Lighting some sandalwood incense or diffusing sandalwood oil will help create a peaceful ambiance. Dab some of the Clear Mind and Vision Blend (p. 126) or sandalwood oil onto your ring finger and gently rub it in the space between your brows. Collect your brow chakra stones and hold them in one hand to help facilitate your visualization meditation, or place them nearby for energetic support.

1. Lie down and close your eyes.

2. Take a deep breath in through your nose, exhale out through your mouth, and sigh. Let your muscles soften and your body relax. Repeat this as many times as needed until you feel relaxed and ready for meditation.

3. During your cleansing inhalations and exhalations, as you inhale, visualize your breath as a beautiful indigo light entering in through the space between your brows. With each exhalation, see that light entering into your head and swirling around your brain.

4. Keeping your eyes closed, take a few moments to bring your attention to the energetic and physical space behind your brows, focusing once again on the indigo light that fills that space. Visualize a blue five-pointed star slowly emerging from that indigo light. Observe it carefully, noticing the color, size, and any other details. Look at its dimensions and whether it is spinning or static. Make a mental note of any feelings or thoughts that come to mind as you look at this star, which represents your brow chakra. In particular, notice anything that might tell you about any imbalances or blockages your brow chakra may have or what you may need to do in order to bring it into harmonious balance.

5. Once you feel you have obtained sufficient insight into the functioning of your brow chakra, take a moment to acknowledge and give gratitude to this energy point in your body, and then gently open your eyes.

❧ BROW CHAKRA ACTIVATION

It is helpful to have some indigo-colored items (e.g., a cushion, throw blanket, or clothing) as well as your brow chakra stones and the Clear Mind and Vision Blend (p. 126) or other brow chakra oils around you, as you will be using these to assist in the opening and balancing of the sixth chakra. Before you start the activation, dab some of your custom oil blend or your preferred brow chakra essential oil onto a polished brow chakra stone.

1. This activation can be performed in any comfortable position (standing, lying down, seated), but you do want your head and neck to feel supported, so take that into consideration when choosing your position.

2. Once you are comfortable, close your eyes and take a few moments to get settled, focusing on breathing slowly and fully. With every inhalation and exhalation, feel the muscles soften and loosen in your head and particularly around your forehead.

3. Take the smooth polished stone dipped in the essential oil blend and gently rub it into the space between your brows to activate your third eye.

4. Bringing your attention to your third eye, visualize your breath as a bright indigo light energizing this powerful energy center so you can feel its power. Bring your mind's eye to the five-pointed star, the symbol of the third eye, and visualize it within that indigo light. With each inhalation and exhalation, see the indigo star getting bigger and brighter until it fills your entire head and brain.

5. See this indigo star clearing away any excess mental clutter and making space for your higher self to be heard so you can think from a grounded and centered place, balancing logic and intuition and allowing yourself to honor both facts and feelings.

6. Allow yourself to feel a sense of clarity and confidence in your mind and in your ability to know your truth—to hear it and to act upon it. Embrace this star as your intuitive third eye, which will help you see what is unseen and to connect wisdom from a higher source.

7. With every breath, see that star expanding from your head into your entire body and feel your entire energy body being infused with your innate wisdom and ability to think and act with discernment, always honoring your personal truth and being divinely guided. Take a deep breath and gently open your eyes when you are finished.

✿ BROW CHAKRA REFLECTION

Smudge your sacred space, and wave your smudge stick gently around your head to clear your mind of any unnecessary thoughts or feelings. Take a few drops of your Clear Mind and Vision Blend (p. 126) or vetiver oil and massage it gently onto your temples and the space between your brows. You may also want to breathe in your blend to connect to the energetic properties.

Now turn to your journal and jot down any reflections you may have on the Brow Chakra Visualization and Activation. Consider what you have learned about your third eye chakra, particularly whether you have experienced any imbalances and any symptoms of this chakra being unbalanced. Make a note of any other intuitive insights you may have regarding the energies of the brow chakra. Also take note of what else you may need to do in order to ensure you are able to think with clarity and confidence, trusting your inner voice and operating from your higher self. Use these questions to guide your reflection:

- Do you trust your inner wisdom?
- Do you trust the wisdom of others?
- Are you discerning? And how do you discern who and what are for your highest good?
- Do you take the time to cultivate your mind to continue to learn?
- Do you have a clear vision for your life? Are you confident in that vision knowing it reflects your truth?
- Can you accept that sometimes you can know things without needing facts or evidence, just from your feelings?

- Do you have a healthy sense of boundaries?
- Can you see that what is right for others and what is their truth may not necessarily be your truth?

❀ BROW CHAKRA AFFIRMATIONS

Brow chakra affirmations should be repeated multiple times a day when going through the opening and aligning process. These affirmations are also helpful when you need to balance the logical and intuitive sides of your brain, and when you need to consider decisions from an even perspective that reflects your innate wisdom, faith, and pragmatism.

Begin by inhaling one of the brow chakra essential oils, either by sniffing it or using a steam inhalation. Dab some of the Clear Mind and Vision Blend or another brow chakra oil of your choice, such as patchouli, in the space between your brows. Stand or sit tall, dropping your shoulders, lifting your head high, and straightening your neck. As you repeat each mantra on the following page, visualize a bright indigo light entering into your third eye and permeating your entire head and brain. Allow this light to infuse you with clarity and connection to your own intuition and divine guidance.

- I know the importance of having a clear mind so I can follow my innate wisdom.

- I take regular steps to declutter my mind of thoughts and feelings that don't serve me and stop me from tapping into my inner guidance.

- I know that my true self is wise, intuitive, and discerning.

- I embrace and trust my inner wisdom and guidance.

- I balance facts with feelings and hope with pragmatism.

- I trust myself and believe in my ability to create the life that I desire.

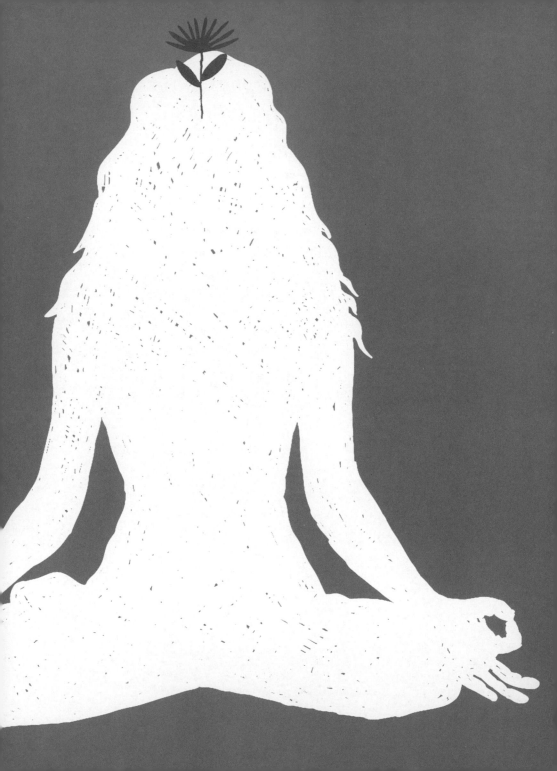

EIGHT

CROWN CHAKRA

**WITH OUR DIVINE CONNECTION
WE ARE ALWAYS IN TOUCH WITH
THE SOLUTIONS WE ARE SEEKING.**

Wayne Dyer

The crown chakra is the seventh and final primary energy point in the body. As its name suggests, this chakra is found at the crown of the head. The Sanskrit name of the crown chakra is Sahasrara, which translates to "thousand petal lotus"; thus, the crown chakra is considered the seat of consciousness.

This sacred seventh and final main energy center governs the entirety of our consciousness—our thoughts, wisdom, and awareness, as well as our connection to the universe and the divine. This chakra's traits include unity, enlightenment, serenity, and the ability to see the beauty (essentially the divine) in everything. Whereas the root, being the first of the chakras, deals with our physical realities and our connection to earthly life, the crown governs our spiritual existence and our connection to both the universe and the higher realm of the divine. The Sahasrara also plays a fundamental role in the functioning of our energy bodies, as it regulates the dispersion of prana (life force energy) into the six other chakras located below the crown. The seventh chakra is often seen as the bridge between the physical and nonphysical realms.

CROWN CHAKRA IMBALANCE

Since this chakra governs our spiritual connection and our consciousness, and because it plays such a crucial role in the health of the other chakras, it is imperative that it be open and balanced for the overall healthy functioning of our energy bodies. In the case of a blocked or underactive crown chakra, we are likely to feel apathetic, lonely, passive, energetically numb, and physically fatigued. We may be disconnected from others (emotionally and otherwise) or have a lack of direction, which results in being unable to establish or manifest our goals. There can be a sense of aimlessly drifting through life without purpose or connection.

Often, an overactive crown chakra results in a desire for material belongings, which can never be satisfied. This greed and superficiality can also manifest as arrogance about life, which extends to others, resulting in a further disconnect from humanity. Instead of seeing the divine connection among all of us, we see only what disconnects us from others. A spiritual disconnect from the divine is a disconnect from all that is—both other beings and the universe.

CORRESPONDENCES

COLOR	ELEMENT	SYMBOL	SHAPE
Violet	The Cosmos		A circular, half-moon shape

PLANET	ASTROLOGICAL SIGNS
The Universe	None (transcends the zodiac)

STONES		GODDESS ARCHETYPE
Selenite	Amethyst	The Guru
Clear quartz	Diamond	

ANIMAL	ESSENTIAL OILS	
Eagle	Lavender	Myrrh
	Frankincense	Spikenard

However, there is such a thing as too much of a good thing—and an overactive crown chakra can be detrimental in multiple ways. It can lead to us being obsessive in our spirituality. We may need a spiritual fix in order to get through our day, which is unhealthy when used as a crutch, much like cigarettes. (Addictions are addictions!) We can also become very ungrounded as we pursue our divine connection at the cost of our earthly life, forgetting the very important anchor of our root chakra. We may find ourselves constantly on the lookout for signs from the divine and believing or overanalyzing everything we see or experience.

I experienced this firsthand a few years into my spiritual awakening when I pursued my divine knowledge and connection in an ungrounded, bordering on obsessive, manner at the expense of practicalities and my physical life. I believe experiencing an overactive crown chakra happens to most people at some point during their spiritual awakening; however, it is important to be aware of this and not float off into the cosmos at the cost of life on Earth.

The seventh energy center governs the pineal glands and our neurological system as well as our eyes, ears, and nose. Common physical ailments due to a blocked brow chakra include the following:

- Migraines
- Pituitary gland issues
- Thyroid issues

- Hormonal imbalances

- Chronic fatigue

- Hair loss

- Cognitive issues

- Neurological disorders

- Nerve pain

- Psychological issues, from anxiety to depression

WHEN THE CROWN CHAKRA OPENS

As with all the chakras, there are some uncomfortable symptoms, both physically and mentally, as this energy center opens. With the crown chakra, you may feel some intense sensations at the top of your head, typically a tingling, which can lead to a more powerful vibration that can make the skull, head, body, and nerves throb. In some cases, you may feel an intense pressure as this energy center opens, resulting in headaches, dizziness, disorientation, a ringing in the ears or head, or a mild feeling of electric energy as though you are being zapped!

During the alignment of the crown chakra, you are likely to experience an increased sense of intuition and connection to both yourself and the spiritual realm. Whether you consider the divine to be God, angels, the universe, or spirit animals—however you define it—you are likely to feel this powerful connection. As you experience this connection, you may have a surge of emotions and feel more attached to others while perhaps simultaneously realizing your detachment from them (especially in the case of an underactive crown chakra). More pleasant symptoms include unity with all of existence and a sense of bliss and peace from knowing that there is more than just what we experience on Earth. You see beauty in all things, and as a result, appreciate your own beauty, not just in your physical self but in your spiritual self. A bonus is that your inner beauty now radiates externally.

During this experience, it is also normal to feel some of the old overactive or underactive symptoms temporarily rearing their head again, but this is usually just a temporary part of the process of alignment. You may find that as a result of your crown chakra opening, you feel a flood of energy both physically and spiritually coursing across your body, and the other chakras may awaken further or go through a natural balancing process.

GODDESS ARCHETYPE: THE GURU

The Guru is the spiritual teacher, showing students how to live in a spiritually enlightened manner. Of course, there are many different teachers across religions and spiritual circles, but what sets the Guru apart is that she is able to impart divine wisdom, the desire for self-realization, and a sense of wholeness within her students. This Guru doesn't want to be your Guru; she wants you to be your own Guru. The Guru wants to see her students both become the very best version of themselves through their divine connection and rise above the earthly physical plane, beyond the material and worldly life.

In some ways, the Guru can resemble the Wise Woman (p. 120), the goddess archetype of the brow chakra, but whereas the Wise Woman is indeed wise, the Guru is divinely wise. The Guru sees all and knows the divine connection between every event and the purpose of even those that seem bad.

Just as the crown chakra is at the top of the chakra ladder, the Guru is the head archetype of the chakra system, making her a role model for each and every one of us. However, this doesn't make the pure Guru arrogant or hierarchical. In fact, a truly powerful Guru knows that because everyone and everything is connected, every-one is also a teacher and lessons come from all life experiences, good and bad.

The Guru represents the spiritual teacher that resides in each of us, in our higher selves. We may not think of ourselves as ever being enlightened enough to become a Guru, and perhaps we will never be spiritual teachers, but that does not mean we can't adopt the traits of the Guru and use them as a role model for the development of our crown chakra. Our ultimate goal in our chakra work is to reach this level of enlightenment, much like the Guru, and to realize that we are more than this earth and this body, that there is so much more to us and our existence, that everything is connected, and ultimately that we are one. It is then that we see there is beauty in everything.

The opening of the crown chakra, despite its odd sensations, was one of my favorite experiences and a turning point for me, as I realized I no longer needed a specific Guru or spiritual teacher. Instead, I knew that all of life would be my teacher. I couldn't conceive of it at the time, but I became a spiritual teacher myself. However, the truth is that as much as I am a teacher, I am more so an eternal student of life.

CROWN CHAKRA STONES

Some of my favorite stones for the crown chakra are recommended here. The majority are colorless, and I find this both calming and a reminder of the pure divine energy of this energy center.

SELENITE

A clear, colorless stone, selenite is exceptionally vibrational, distilling negative emotions and bringing clarity to the mind. This ethereal stone connects us to our higher consciousness and to the realm of the divine, so it's wonderful to use for opening the crown chakra. Selenite wands carry a very purifying energy and can clear the aura of both people and items. I use mine to clear crystals and other items I keep in my sacred space for ritual and meditation.

CLEAR QUARTZ

One of my must-have stones is clear quartz. This common yet extraordinary stone has powerful cleansing and energizing properties. I like to use both polished clear quartz stones and wands for meditation, rituals, and healing. Placing a medium-sized polished clear quartz stone on top of one's head or surrounding the head area during the Crown Chakra Activation (p. 148) will help open this powerful energy center and facilitate a divine connection.

DIAMOND

Diamonds are not only a girl's best friend but also a powerful stone for our healing tool kit. Often referred to as the Stone of Invincibility, thanks to its hard nature, diamonds have purifying, protective, courageous, and abundant energies. You can use a piece of diamond jewelry during your crown chakra meditations and rituals, and then wear it with the intention for it to continue to stimulate your divine connection.

AMETHYST

Amethyst is a wonderful stone for meditation and rituals and for balancing all the chakras. In relation to the crown chakra, it is best to try and obtain an amethyst crystal that is as indigo as possible to tap into the seventh chakra. By using amethyst in ritual or meditation, you can bring tranquility to your mind and clear it so you can experience the pure consciousness, wisdom, and bliss that come with a fully open and balanced crown chakra. I have a large piece of raw amethyst on my altar, and I use some small tumbled amethyst stones in meditation, ritual, and healing sessions.

CROWN CHAKRA ESSENTIAL OILS

All of the essential oils recommended here have calming and relaxing properties, and some also have a mystical connotation. (Frankincense and myrrh were considered to be gifts fit for a king, as referred to in the biblical story of the three wise men.)

LAVENDER

Just as amethyst serves as a healing stone for all seven of the chakras, so too is lavender oil universal in its energetic assistance to all of the chakras. When it comes to the crown chakra, lavender brings calmness and peace of mind, which facilitates clear-mindedness and maintains the open and balanced flow of the seventh energy center. Diffusing this oil for rituals and meditation or placing a few drops on your pillow at night promotes peace of mind and a divine connection.

FRANKINCENSE

Often referred to as the holy oil, frankincense is another must-have in your essential oil toolbox, as it promotes tranquility and activates a spiritual connection. You can diffuse this oil for meditation and rituals or take a few direct inhalations to create an almost instant energetic shift. This ancient oil has certain properties that stimulate the pineal and pituitary glands, so it has both emotional and physical benefits. I like to diffuse frankincense oil by itself and combine it with other oils to create a custom blend.

SPIKENARD

A lesser known but potent essential oil, spikenard has a rich, earthy aroma that is grounding and can balance an overactive crown chakra. This oil also has properties that help the brain and relieve some tension headaches and migraines that are symptomatic of an imbalanced seventh chakra. I like to diffuse this oil along with frankincense if I am feeling tense or my head feels cloudy.

MYRRH

Another mystical essential oil, myrrh is wonderful for stimulating an underactive or blocked crown chakra. I recommend using this oil as part of a custom blend for massaging the scalp and helping to open the crown chakra.

DIVINE CONNECTION BLEND

The purpose of this custom oil blend is to connect you to your higher self and the divine realm. The energies of the divine connection blend will assist with rituals and meditation during the process of opening and balancing the crown chakra. You can also use this blend at times when you feel disconnected from yourself, others, or the universe, or when you need a little energetic assistance to reconnect to your spiritual path.

INGREDIENTS

2 tbsp almond oil (or other carrier oil)
3 drops lavender essential oil
2 drops frankincense essential oil
2 drops myrrh essential oil
1 drop spikenard essential oil

TOOLS/EQUIPMENT

2 oz. dark glass bottle
Dropper

YIELD

Makes 1.5 oz.

1. Pour the almond oil into a dark glass bottle.

2. Using a dropper, add each essential oil. Cover the bottle and swirl lightly.

3. Massage or dab the oil onto the top of your head and neck or inhale directly as needed. (For external use only.)

☖ CROWN CHAKRA VISUALIZATION

To best facilitate this meditation, it is important to cleanse the physical and energetic space of the crown chakra. Take a few moments to smudge your space and self. You can take your sage bundle and gently wave it around the crown of your head. Another powerful way to do this is take some of the Divine Connection Blend (p. 146) or frankincense oil and massage it onto the top of your head using a medium-sized polished crown chakra stone, such as clear quartz or selenite. Diffuse lavender oil or another of the crown chakra oils. Take a few deep inhalations of these oils, then settle into a comfortable position.

1. Lie down and close your eyes. Take a few cleansing breaths, inhaling through your nostrils and exhaling out of your mouth while visualizing your breath as a beautiful violet light.

2. Bring your attention to the crown of your head and see your breath as a vibrant violet light entering into your head and flooding your entire head and brain. See the violet light wafting in all the parts of your head and feel its soft, pure energy.

3. Focus on the crown of your head and see the violet light forming a half moon on top of your head, symbolizing

your crown chakra. Notice what this half moon looks and feels like; observe its exact shape, dimensions, and color and whether it is static or spinning. Continuing to observe this half moon, make a mental note of any images that come to mind, memories, feelings, thoughts, and intuitive insights you receive as to the state of this powerful energy center.

4. Once you feel you have obtained sufficient insight into the functioning of your crown chakra, take a moment to acknowledge and give gratitude to this energy point in your body, and then gently open your eyes.

꧁ CROWN CHAKRA ACTIVATION

Massage your scalp with a few drops of the Divine Connection Blend (p. 146) or a crown chakra oil. Then take a shower and wash your hair thoroughly, massaging the crown of your head gently and visualizing the water purifying both your physical and energetic bodies. This activation is best performed with the assistance of natural light. You can be outdoors, elements permitting, but if you prefer to be inside, carry out the activation near a window or in a room with natural light. Have your crown chakra stones in hand. If you have selenite or quartz wands, wave them around the top of your head to help clear it energetically.

1. Take one of your smooth, polished crown chakra stones and place it on the crown of your head as though you are wearing a crystal cap. Focusing on the crown of your head, visualize once again the violet half moon and see the healing violet light permeate through your entire head and brain. Feel the healing and calming qualities of this light and start to breathe more consciously.

2. As you breathe in, call in clarity, expanded conscious- ness, and divine connection. As you exhale, release thoughts that do not serve you or that are outdated, disharmonious, or unloving.

3. Bring your attention to the violet half moon crowning your head and see an opening at the top of it, which allows light to stream in. See this light as a purifying golden light. With your breath, inhale this light through the opening of the half moon and see it shining into your head, almost like a torchlight. Welcome this light as your divine connection, which allows you to connect to both your higher self and the divine realm.

4. Feel a sense of peace and expansion within your mind and a realization that everything and everyone is connected. There is divine order in your life, even if it

does not appear so. Feel a sense of gratitude flood your body as you realize the connection and beauty in all of existence.

5. Focusing once again on the crown of your head, see the violet half moon transform into a beautiful violet lotus, which starts to open up with more petals than you can count, all opening up toward that golden light, which continues to emanate from above.

6. As this lotus continues to flower, feel a sensation of calm flood your entire body from head to toe as you realize that you are divinely connected, guided, and protected. Gently open your eyes when you are finished.

❀ CROWN CHAKRA REFLECTION

Settling into your sacred space or another chosen spot, light some palo santo or diffuse palo santo oil. If you have a selenite or quartz wand, wave it around your head. Take a few drops of your Divine Connection Blend (p. 146) or lavender oil and rub it in your hands; cup your hands to inhale the blend. Place an amethyst crystal on your writing desk or wherever you are seated. Take one of your polished stones and hold it in your hands for a few moments, connecting to its clarifying properties.

Journal about your Crown Chakra Visualization and Activation. Note what you have learned so far about your crown chakra and any insights you may have on how you can bring this powerful energy center into alignment and optimal flow. Use these questions as a guide for your reflection:

- Do you view your life experiences through a spiritual perspective?

- What is your spiritual truth(s), and do you honor this in your life?

- Do you engage in religious and/or spiritual rituals, and do you do these with intention?

- Do you feel connected to yourself and a higher source when conducting rituals?

- Do you appreciate the beauty of nature?

- Are you able to see that an appreciation of beauty, whether in yourself, others, or nature, makes life more enjoyable?

- Do you believe it's your birthright to experience bliss?

- Do you feel that you need to solve all your problems or achieve certain things to experience deep happiness?

- Are you comfortable with stillness and silence?

- Do you feel connected to yourself and all living beings, whether people, animals, or plants?

✿ CROWN CHAKRA AFFIRMATIONS

Crown chakra affirmations provide support when you are in the process of opening and aligning this energy center. By repeating them multiple times a day, you can create a mental, emotional, and energetic shift that will facilitate the opening and balanced flow of the seventh chakra. You can also repeat these whenever you need to embody more of the traits of the Guru and the positive qualities of a balanced crown chakra. These mantras are best repeated silently with your eyes closed.

To begin, diffuse one or a combination of your crown chakra essential oils, and inhale the aroma deeply. Dab some of your Divine Connection Blend (p. 146), or another crown chakra oil, on the top of your head, your temples, and the back of your neck. Focusing your attention on the crown of your head, visualize the violet half moon once more. Begin to repeat your affirmations, and as you do so, envision a violet light swirling around your half moon. Allow this light to infuse you with calmness, and the knowledge that all is well and as it should be. As you repeat your affirmations, see the violet half moon slowly transform into a beautiful lotus flower, and as the flower opens, feel a sense of peace, connection, and utter bliss flood your body.

- I am one with the universe.
- I am one with the Divine.

- I honor and nurture my divine connection.
- I embrace the perfection in imperfection.
- I trust that all that is unfolding is for my highest good.
- I am at peace with myself, others, and all of life.
- I experience bliss regularly, simply from living my everyday life.

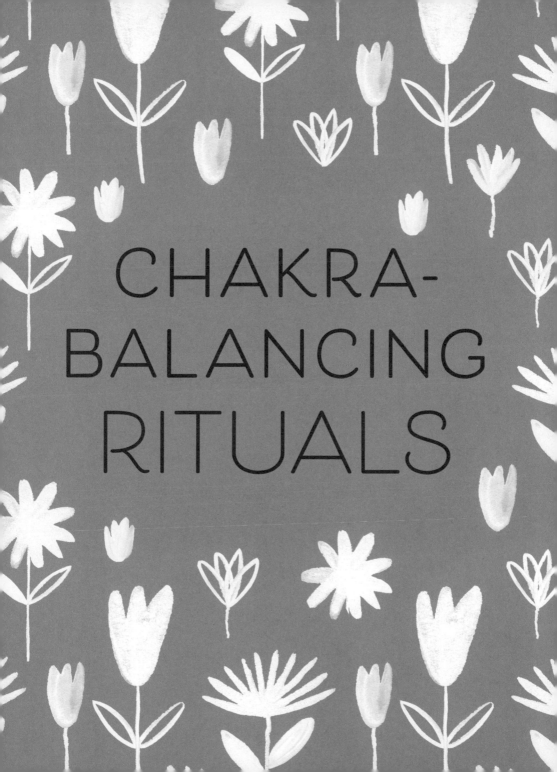

CHAKRA-BALANCING RITUALS

NINE

SIMPLE DAILY RITUALS

ANY RITUAL IS AN OPPORTUNITY FOR TRANSFORMATION.

Starhawk

As you are now aware, how we spend our days, the environments we are in, the energies we are subjected to, the conversations we have, and the situations we have to navigate all impact us physically and energetically—in our mind, body, and soul. As a result, a spoke in the energetic wheels of our body can break at any time. Even after we've opened and balanced our chakras, it doesn't mean that daily life won't throw us off-kilter. Thankfully, there are many rituals that can help us to navigate the flow of our day and help us keep our energy levels clear and aligned.

CREATING NEW RITUALS

You may have heard the saying that it is not what we do now and then that counts but what we do daily that positively affects our lives. However, for the majority of us, our daily lives are often more of a daily grind. We have jobs to maintain, housework to complete, and children, pets, and other family members to care for. We may find ourselves wearing so many hats and doing so much multitasking that even the basics of taking care of ourselves, like eating breakfast, often fall by the wayside.

Your morning may go something like this: You get out of bed late, feel anxious as you have to rush to get ready for work, forget breakfast, and then caffeinate to make up for it. You tend to those who rely on you and feel irritated by them. You check your phone and scroll through a series of stress-inducing headlines or social media feeds that make you feel unsettled, and then battle rush-hour traffic filled with other similarly stressed-out commuters, all before getting to work to face a challenging situation with a coworker or boss. It's not even 9:00 a.m., and most of your energy body is already out of whack! This is, sadly, too familiar for most of us. I spent many years operating like this and told myself, as I am sure you are probably telling yourself, that this was just life. What I didn't realize is how much of my routine was made up of bad habits that had become daily rituals.

Think of all the unconscious rituals we have: brushing our teeth, pouring our morning cup of joe, and scrolling on our phones. And then imagine how we can consciously create rituals. Rest assured, it isn't as difficult as you may imagine, nor is it time-consuming or expensive. Self-care may seem like a luxury and an indulgence you can't possibly afford. It may feel as though it's for those who don't work or have responsibilities, or for those who have endless funds. But daily self-care doesn't have to be complicated or expensive.

Beginning your day with a simple self-care ritual, like the five-minute Energy Activation (p. 162), means you'll be starting off on the right foot, mentally and physically. And as your day goes on, you can do check-ins to anchor yourself, clear your energy, connect to your breath, or do meditatations, like the Grounding Breath (p. 169) or Brain-Balancing Breath (p. 171) rituals. You will notice the day-to-day difference in how they assist you, but what is more important is how they play a powerful role in the bigger picture of your life.

Rituals can be acts of caring for ourselves with mindful intention, powerful acts of self-love. These daily acts of self-care foster a greater connection to our higher selves, others, and nature. They can help us feel safe and balanced, regardless of what is happening in the world. Rituals also help us take responsibility for our lives and remind us that we are the co-creators of our lives and not simply subjects to the daily tides. Plus, as you will see, they can become a really enjoyable part of your daily routine and your lifestyle.

STAYING ON COURSE

We know the importance of rituals, but as the saying goes, the road to hell is paved with good intentions. Just because we know something is good for us doesn't necessarily mean it is easy for us to do it. We all know going to the gym and exercising regularly will improve our health, but how many times have we paid for a gym membership and left it unused?

Inspiration gets us started, but habit is what keeps us going. We must make our rituals daily habits written into our day, like eating meals or brushing our teeth. We don't skip these, but the truth is that even with the best intentions, we may end up skipping our morning meditation or deciding we don't have time for it on a given day because life threw a curveball our way. Perhaps, like me, you are a mother with a baby and wake up early to meditate before the baby is up, but the baby decides to wake up midway through your meditation, so you put it off until later, but then it doesn't happen. You say to yourself, "I am a mother. I don't have time for this meditating stuff at this stage of my life." However, the truth is you do have time for it, and if you're like me, you need it more than ever.

KEEPING DAILY RITUALS

The truth is that everyone has five minutes a day to meditate or to practice a ritual. Obstacles pop up, babies wake up, life gets busy, we wake up late, we are rushing, someone in our life has a crisis and needs us. Every day something can happen to take us away from our rituals, and every day we need to put our hands back on our hearts and remind ourselves of the powerful role our energy bodies play in our well-being. We need to have the discipline to carry out our rituals and ingrain these rituals into our daily lives, so they become as everyday as brushing our teeth. Here are some tips for keeping our rituals:

- **PLAN.** You can plan out your rituals according to your day and/or week. Scheduling in your rituals makes it more likely you will do them.

- **BE FLEXIBLE.** If you didn't do your morning meditation, that doesn't mean you don't do it at all. You can just do it later.

- **PERSONALIZE IT.** I offer multiple rituals in this book, but they don't need to be rigidly adhered to. The most important thing is that the rituals work for you, so feel free to tweak and personalize them.

- **JOIN FORCES.** You can team up with a friend, co-worker, or loved one for some of your rituals. Even if you don't do them together, you can be each other's ritual support buddies!

- **BE PATIENT.** Change doesn't happen overnight. You need to carry out rituals consistently for some time before you can truly enjoy their benefits.

❀ ENERGY ACTIVATION RITUAL

BEST TIME OF DAY:
Morning or when you need an energetic lift

TIME:
5 minutes

This Energy Activation Ritual is a powerful way of creating an almost instant boost in energy levels. Ideally you would undertake this ritual first thing in the morning, so your day starts with and maintains this positive vibe; however, if you're unable do it first thing in the morning, you can always do it later in the day or as needed.

1. Set the intention to receive the energetic shift and boost you need to be your best self.

2. Stand tall with your feet planted firmly on the ground beneath you, ideally with your shoes off (you can keep your socks on).

3. Drop your shoulders, straighten your neck, and lift your head high.

4. Breathing into your navel, as you exhale, visualize your breath as a bright yellow light entering your belly and then permeating your entire body. Using your intention and mind's eye, see and feel this yellow light as a powerful life-force energy.

5. As you breathe in this vibrant life-force energy, envision it stimulating every cell, bone, muscle, and tissue in your body. Visualize this life force coursing through your body, energizing you physically, mentally, emotionally, and spiritually. Feel uplifted, vibrant, and ready for the day.

6. Giving thanks to this vibrant life-force energy that you can always tap into and utilize. Take a few deep inhalations through your nose, exhale loudly through your mouth, and sigh to seal this ritual.

✿ PROTECTIVE SHIELD VISUALIZATION

BEST TIME OF DAY:
Morning

TIME:
5 minutes

We are energy beings who are affected by other energies, but we can't control third parties or external events. What we *can* do is take precautionary measures to preserve our energy bodies from negative external influences. This meditation is best performed standing or seated. I recommend doing this before you leave your house or when you feel the need for a protective shield around your aura. I used to do it regularly on the Tube when I lived in London!

1. Whether you are standing or seated, plant your feet firmly on the ground and feel your connection to the earth, visualizing roots coming up from deep in Earth's core through the surface upon which your feet are resting and into the soles of your feet. Take a few deep breaths, continuing this visualization and focusing on your connection to the earth and feeling grounded with each breath.

2. Drop and relax your shoulders, allowing your neck and head to relax.

3. Bring your attention to the top of your head. Using your breath, visualize that you are breathing into a small opening at the crown of your head and that this breath is a golden light that is shining down from the skies through the building or place where you are situated and entering the crown of your head. Feel your connection to the divine realm and the cosmos with each breath and visualization.

4. Using your mind's eye, visualize a transparent bubble or sphere around yourself. Use your imagination and creativity. The most important thing is to feel and see this as your protective energy shield, visible and known only to you. See it surrounding you, and see yourself within this sphere, knowing that all that happens outside of this sphere is not yours to act on. Feel a sense of relief and gratitude as you see this bubble surrounding you, protecting you, and preserving your energy field.

5. Open your eyes and continue with your day, still keeping that vision of the energy bubble in your mind's eye.

✿ DAILY BRAIN DUMP

BEST TIME OF DAY:
Morning or evening

TIME
15 minutes

Most of us live in our heads. We have too many thoughts filling our minds, which can create energetic imbalances and cause us emotional discomfort. Our minds become full rather than mindful. In the same way that we go to the bathroom every day and let go of the excess waste from our body, we need to also let go of the excess thoughts filling our mind. To begin, light a scented candle or incense stick or diffuse an essential oil. Set aside a journal dedicated to your daily brain dumps, and remember that this is a journal for releasing thoughts into, not for reflecting on them.

1. Open your journal and write for 15 minutes. It doesn't matter what you write; it doesn't matter if it doesn't make sense. It doesn't matter if it's illegible. If you don't know what to write, you can simply write, "I don't know what to write," for three pages! Write without censorship or trying to be perfect.

2. Once you've written for approximately 15 minutes or three pages, close your journal and light some palo santo.

3. Take a few deep inhalations, and put away your journal.

❀ MINDFUL MANIFESTING VISUALIZATION

BEST TIME OF DAY:
Morning

TIME:
5 to 10 minutes

So often we live our lives subconsciously, without intention. The Mindful Manifesting Visualization simply requires you to set intentions as to how you want your day to go based on how you want to feel during or at the end of the day. All that is required is your intention and imagination!

1. Think of three things you wish to happen today, and set intentions for them.

2. Now begin to visualize your ideal day in detail and how you feel as a result. What happens first in your desired day, and how does it make you feel? Continue with this process of visualizing and experiencing each stage of the manifestation of the day you desire.

3. Get passionate as you use your intention and mind's eye to visualize and create those feelings flooding your body.

4. Take a few deep cleansing breaths, imagining you are breathing in and out of your heart center, and feel that sense of happiness in your heart at the prospect of manifesting and enjoying the day you desire.

✿ DAILY AFFIRMATIONS

**BEST TIME
OF DAY:**
Morning

TIME:
5 to 10
minutes

Affirming the day helps create the day you desire. These Daily Affirmations can be a mixture of the different chakra affirmations. You can create a set of affirmations you wish to repeat each morning and a different set for each evening. You can even put together affirmations you like to repeat to help you get through the day. You can be creative with these and tweak or add to them as you need.

Affirmations are usually spoken out loud, but if necessary, you can repeat these silently in your head. You can also write down your affirmations if needed or if that serves you better. However you choose to perform your affirmations, do so with passion and conviction, believing in your words and feeling them as you speak or write them. For extra effectiveness and connection, you can repeat these while looking into your own eyes with a mirror.

✿ GROUNDING BREATH MEDITATION

BEST TIME OF DAY:
Midday

TIME:
5 minutes

We become ungrounded daily due to the busyness, stresses, and strains of everyday life. When this happens, we often find ourselves feeling spacey, as we are disconnected from our bodies. By connecting to our breath, we reconnect to our bodies and, in turn, ground ourselves, which promotes a feeling of safety and connection. This is a great midday or afternoon ritual to connect you to your breath and ground you.

1. Find a quiet and pleasant spot to sit or stand and conduct this breathing.

2. Close your eyes and turn inward, becoming aware of your breath. Notice its quality: Is it shallow or deep? Does it feel measured or frantic? Observe the quality of your breath without judging it.

3. Bring your attention to your feet and plant them firmly on the ground, really feeling them and their connection to the earth.

CONTINUED ▶▶

4. Slowing down your breath, inhale deeply, visualizing your breath as coming up from the center of Earth, through the roots beneath the surface of the ground you are on, and finally entering into your body.

5. As you exhale, visualize your breath flooding your body and then going down through the soles of your feet, into the roots beneath the ground, and deep into Earth's core.

6. As you continue this breath visualization, really feel your body connect to Earth. Repeat silently, "I am connected, I am safe, I am grounded."

7. After several breaths and once you feel sufficiently grounded, gently open your eyes.

❀ BRAIN-BALANCING BREATH MEDITATION

BEST TIME OF DAY:
Midday

TIME:
5 minutes

As we go about our daily lives and perform our duties, whether professional or personal, we can experience an imbalance between the right and left hemispheres of our brain. As a result, our divine feminine energy, which promotes intuition and creativity, becomes blocked. This simple breathing exercise helps bring peace of mind and clarity as well as balance to both sides of the brain. It can be particularly useful when you are going from a task that requires more of the logical/practical side of your brain to one that requires the creative/intuitive side (e.g., when you finish your day job and want to work on your creative side project or do spiritual work.)

1. Find a comfortable spot where you can relax and perform this exercise.

CONTINUED ▶▶

2. Use your right thumb to close your right nostril, and then inhale through your left nostril. Use your right ring finger to close your left nostril, then lift your right thumb off your nose, and exhale through your right nostril.

3. Repeat in opposite order. Inhale through your right nostril, then use your thumb to close the right nostril, and release the left nostril to exhale through your left nostril. This represents one cycle.

4. Repeat this cycle ten times.

5. Once you are finished, take a few deep inhalations through both nostrils, and exhale and sigh out of your mouth.

CHAKRA OPENING AND BALANCING MEDITATION

BEST TIME OF DAY: Evening

TIME: 35 minutes

Elements of this meditation may remind you of the chakra visualization or activation exercises from earlier chapters. The purpose of this meditation is to provide a shorter opening and balancing activity for the entire energy body. Perform this every week on Sunday evenings to make sure your chakras are open and spinning for the week ahead. Before you begin, prepare your sacred space by smudging and clearing the energy, diffusing lavender essential oil or lighting a sandalwood incense stick, and collecting your polished clear quartz or selenite stones.

1. Lie down in a comfortable position, either holding your stones in your hands or placing them nearby.
2. Take a few deep inhalations through your nose, and exhale through your mouth. With every breath, feel your body relax, all the muscles softening and loosening as you sink deeper into the surface you are lying on.

CONTINUED ▶▶

3. Using your mind's eye, start to scan your body from the tip of your toes through to the top of your head. Notice what you see and how each part of the body feels.

4. As you scan the physical location of each chakra, pause and focus on the color related to this energy wheel. Using your breath and intention, visualize the color as a gentle light that grows and spins as you activate and bring balance to this energy center. Take your time to work through each of the chakras using this visualization to both activate and bring balance.

5. You may find that during this process some of your chakras require more time and focus than others. This is a sign as to which ones are experiencing more imbalances than others.

6. Make a mental note of any observations, visuals, or feelings that come to mind as you conduct this exercise, and jot them down once you have finished with the meditation.

✿ RELEASE LIST RITUAL

BEST TIME OF DAY:
Evening

TIME:
10 minutes

Things happen every week (sometimes daily!) that cause us to feel emotionally off or energetically imbalanced. This Release List Ritual is a cathartic and powerful way of letting go of the things that have caused us to feel off. As you practice this ritual regularly, you will feel a tangible physical, emotional, and energetic release. I once went through an entire month where I conducted this ritual daily! This can be done any time of day, whenever is practical for you to do so, and as many times as needed—though I find it most beneficial to do this in the evening. For extra impact, I follow it up with the Energy Healing Shower Meditation (p. 177).

1. Grab a pen and piece of paper.
2. At the top of the sheet of paper, write down the following (or something similar that suits you):

> *I release all that is written below because it does not serve me or my highest good. By releasing the below, I physically, emotionally, and energetically reset myself.*

CONTINUED ▶▶

3. Below that statement, write down anything that is bothering you (e.g., feeling embarrassed about X, feeling upset about my conversation with X, feeling anger and frustration toward X, feeling fear or worry about X).

4. After you have finished writing your list, read it and take a few deep cleansing breaths as you prepare to destroy it and release the situations and negative energies listed.

5. To destroy the release list, you can burn, shred, or tear it. I find it most cathartic to safely burn my list and watch it go up in flames, feeling the energies of the situations I am releasing leave my body like the smoke of the burning list. However, some people enjoy shredding their list or tearing it up into several pieces. However you choose to get rid of it, make sure you feel a sense of palpable release as you let go of the energies.

6. If you have the time, you can seal this ritual with the Energy Healing Shower Meditation (p. 177). If not, wash your hands and splash your face with some cold water to energetically cleanse and complete this ritual.

❀ ENERGY HEALING SHOWER MEDITATION

BEST TIME OF DAY:
Evening

TIME:
15 to 20 minutes

This shower meditation is a wonderful way of cleansing yourself, both physically and energetically, and can be a very healing experience as you remove any energetic debris from your aura. This is particularly comforting after travel or being in crowded places. Before you start, smudge your bathroom and yourself using a white sage bundle, and diffuse eucalyptus oil.

1. Step into the shower, and let the water pour down on your head and body.

2. With your eyes closed, envision the water as physically cleaning you and energetically washing away anything that did not serve you from your day. See any negativity or stresses leave you, mentally and energetically, as they are washed away. Feel the cleansing and healing energy of the water as it washes you clean and clear, back to your true self.

CONTINUED ▶▶

3. Open your eyes and continue with your usual shower routine. As you wash your body with soap and wash your hair, continue with the intention and visualization of being washed clean and clear, mentally and energetically.

4. Stand tall once again with your eyes closed, and allow the water from the shower to wash over your head and body. Visualize this water as a gentle golden color, which is healing, rebalancing, and restoring.

5. Finish by moisturizing your body and using a few drops of your Peace of Mind Blend (p. 40) or lavender oil to ground you and seal this process.

❧ CHAKRA-BALANCING BATH

Water is a great healer, and baths are a wonderful way to energetically reset. I recommend having a Chakra-Balancing Bath during the process of opening and balancing a chakra as well as when you feel one of your energy centers needs healing and balancing.

1. Collect your oils and crystals depending on the chakra you are focusing on.
2. Place ½ cup of Epsom salt under the warm running tap of your bath. Salt is a great energetic balancer and, combined with water, is very healing.
3. Place a few of your chakra crystals in the water. Smooth, polished crystals work better.
4. Once your bath is full, add 8 to 10 drops of the essential oils of your choice and mix with your hands.
5. Step into your bath, and set the intention to bring healing and balance to the energy center you are focused on.
6. Breathe in the aroma of the scents, and welcome the energetic support of the crystals. Relax and enjoy your bath.

❀ GRATITUDE REFLECTION

BEST TIME OF DAY:
Night

TIME:
5 minutes

I practice this Gratitude Reflection nightly before I go to bed, so I go to bed feeling happy, which helps me to sleep soundly. You don't need any props or tools for this reflection, just an open and grateful heart.

1. Focus on three things for which you are grateful every day (e.g., people, situations, the roof over your head) and how happy and grateful you are for them. Let that sense of gratitude take over your body, softening and opening your heart and bringing physical pleasure to each part of your being.

2. Now focus on three things that happened that day for which you are grateful. They don't have to be big or dramatic. They can be as simple as getting home safely, eating a nourishing meal, or seeing a rainbow. As you think of those things, allow that sense of gratitude to fill your body with positive, loving energy.

3. Give thanks to the universe and the divine for bringing you all of this good. Feel a sense of peace, gratitude, and deep happiness flood your mind, body, and soul as you settle into sleep with appreciation for all that you have, all that is, and all that's to come.

☸ SPACE-CLEARING RITUAL

**BEST TIME
OF DAY:**
Anytime

TIME:
10 minutes

To clear the energy of your home or a particular room, simply light your sage bundle and smudge around the space you are clearing with the intention to remove energetic debris and create a harmonious energy. Keep the windows closed so that when you are done, you can open them to let out any excess smoke and unwanted energies.

If you are clearing a space that is not your own (e.g., an office space or an airplane or travel space), use your selenite or quartz wand and gently wave it about as you would your sage bundle during a smudging ceremony. As you wave the crystal wand, use your intention to visualize any negative energies dissipating and the wands infusing the space with clear, harmonious energies.

Where possible, diffuse essential oils to help clear the space. You can choose an essential oil or a homemade oil spray with water and a few drops of essential oils to clear any unwanted energies and bring energetic equilibrium.

RITUALS IN THIS CHAPTER

TEN

SEASONAL
RENEWAL RITUALS

I HAVE A KIND OF RESPECT—
A WORSHIPFUL ATTITUDE EVEN—
FOR NATURE AND THE NATURAL
ORDER AND THE COSMOS
AND THE SEASONS.

Sidney Poitier

We don't need to cast aside our modern-day comforts to live more like our ancestors and be in tune with nature. Rather, we can enjoy the benefits of our modern-day existence and live in alignment with the natural cycles and seasons of nature and the moon. We are privileged to have the best of both worlds. We just need to educate ourselves, be prepared to make adjustments to our lives, and create rituals so we can be aligned with the different seasons and moon cycles. All of this will help our health and well-being—mind, body, and soul—and have a positive impact on the flow of our lives.

CHANGING WITH THE SEASONS

While humanity has evolved with many welcome technological, scientific, and medical advancements, we are less connected than ever with the natural rhythms of life and nature. We ignore the cues from nature, the changes in daylight, the waxing and waning of the moon, and the shifts in temperature as we move through the seasons. We often continue with our lives on autopilot. We have our heads down toward our phones and digital devices rather than our eyes up to the skies and the natural environment. This denial of our connection to, and the importance of, nature means we live out of sync with natural rhythms and end up disconnected from ourselves.

In truth, the seasons of nature offer us a blueprint for our lives, allowing us to ebb and flow with the natural rhythms of planet Earth and experience different energies, which help us to live more well-rounded and wholesome lives. The traits of each season serve to teach us about ourselves and the natural process of life; however, when we fight the flow of the seasons, we fall out of alignment with nature and ourselves.

The seasons are split into yin and yang energy. We need a combination of both to have balance. We don't want to be too yin or too yang, as it will create disharmony. Fall and winter are yin seasons, which require us to go inward: to rest, restore, and reconnect with divine feminine energies. In these more passive seasons, our job is to simply be. We are to nourish ourselves, take care of the basics, and tailor our lives to the energies of the season. However, people often complain about fall and winter because the cooler temperatures and darker days seemingly restrict us from our busy lives, perhaps causing some people to believe they are operating less optimally. We may try to go about our business as usual rather than simply be. This is why we see a peak in illness during the fall and winter, and why it's dubbed "cold and flu season." We push against our natural rhythm, often compromising our health.

Spring and summer are yang seasons, when we feel a sense of excitement and energy, experience powerful growth, and connect with masculine energies. We are more active and creative, and birth new versions of ourselves. While we may have personal preferences for seasons, we need to work with the energies of each and respect their role in our living balanced lives, physically and energetically.

Our ancestors looked to the seasons to help them live their lives, understanding that the warmth and high energy of summer, with life blooming, would be followed by the cooler temperatures of fall and cyclical decay. They understood that winter served a purpose for them, and they would prepare for this time during the fall harvest. They also knew that, despite the destruction in nature during winter, Mother Nature would regenerate and, come spring, new life would blossom and summer would bring its dues.

SPRING

The spring equinox represents equal parts day and night and marks the official start of spring with a return to the light after the darkness of winter. It also welcomes milder temperatures and longer days. In the spring, we experience a rebirth of sorts after the hibernation of winter. Just as Mother Nature seems to wake from her winter slumber and the natural world begins to blossom once more, so do we.

It's a time for fresh starts and sweet new beginnings, so it makes sense that during this season you want to have a clean slate for life to blossom. This means clearing out any of the cobwebs from winter and making everything fresh, clean, and ready for the new—hence the popular practice of a spring cleaning, one of my favorite seasonal rituals.

It's good to take advantage of milder temperatures in spring to reconnect with Mother Nature and be outside more regularly for fresh air and light. Start to move your body more and exercise. Eat a little lighter, with lots of seasonal fruits and vegetables from local farmers' markets. Allergy season starts in the spring, but ingesting local honey may help alleviate symptoms.

Spring is the time when we really awaken the sacral and heart chakras. The sacral connects to the abundance of the season, and we come into our own personal power as we are reborn. The heart chakra is strengthened in the spring as we see the beauty all around us and the connectedness of the seasons and all of life.

❀ SPRING EQUINOX RITUAL

CHAKRAS:
Heart, sacral,
and throat

WHEN:
In the days
leading up to
and on the day
of the spring
equinox

TIME:
1 to 1.5 hours
per day

The spring equinox is related to new beginnings, fertility, and birth of all kinds, so it's the perfect time to create space for these new beginnings and to plant the seeds you wish to bloom in the season ahead. As part of your Spring Equinox Ritual, you will be conducting a spring cleaning in the lead-up to the equinox itself to prepare yourself and your space to birth newness and experience the fruitfulness of the season.

BEFORE THE SPRING EQUINOX

1. Go through your home and get rid of clutter. Donate, recycle, or dispose of items responsibly. Do the same for your car.

2. Go through your wardrobe and put away your winter clothes, whether in storage or in the back of your closet. Clean all old, musty items and get them fresh and ready to be worn.

3. Conduct a deep cleaning of your home. This means washing carpets, rugs, curtains, and furniture. Move furniture and dust, wipe, vacuum, and mop the spaces that are often ignored.

CONTINUED ▶▶

4. Change your set of bedding from the warmer winter quilts to a lighter spring cover. Choose a lighter, brighter color.

5. Organize your paperwork for the few months that have passed. Don't keep any old receipts or papers lying around. File or shred them!

ON THE DAY OF THE SPRING EQUINOX

1. Take a Chakra-Balancing Bath (p. 179), using jasmine or ylang-ylang essential oils and polished heart and sacral chakra stones.

2. Draw up a list of new things you would like to birth over this new season and existing things you would like to see bloom. Make a list of affirmations from this list.

3. Conduct a simple meditation where you visualize these desires coming to fruition by using your imagination and being creative, trusting in your power to manifest your desires and feeling the happiness in your heart.

4. Finally, to complete your ritual, speak your affirmations out loud, really using your voice, whether through song or speech, and place your list on your altar along with any items that may represent the manifestation of your desires.

SUMMER

The summer solstice is the longest day of the year with the maximum amount of sunlight and heralds the official start of summer. It represents both a peak in the year and the midpoint, but there is plenty of sunshine to be enjoyed in the months following the solstice. The days slowly endure less sunlight until fall, when there are equal parts sun and moon once again.

Just as summer is the season of the sun, it also represents the fiery energy of our solar plexus chakra, the precious jewel of our personal energy center. It is a highly energized season when we focus on our individual potential to manifest our desires for the rest of the year and are encouraged to connect to the more masculine manifesting energy of the sun. As we enjoy the physical sunlight, we can harness this energy to allow our unique personas to bask in the spotlight.

As the sunny sky radiates warmth, so too do we in this season. When energized by sunlight and longer days, we have more energy to socialize, pursue our passions, and live with confidence and clarity. Summer recharges our personal energy batteries and reminds us of the importance of pleasure and having fun.

Eating lots of seasonal citrus fruits and drinking lots of lemon and ginger water are wonderful ways to work with the energies of summer to keep clear and hydrated. It's also a great time to do more cardio exercise and get your heart rate and endorphins pumping. If you can combine those with the outdoors and sunshine, even better! Just make sure to be well hydrated and use lots of SPF.

☖ SUMMER SOLSTICE RITUAL

CHAKRAS:
Solar plexus
and sacral

WHEN:
On the day of
the summer
solstice

TIME:
1 hour

At the summer solstice, we experience the greatest amount of daylight as we embrace the start of summer. Just as we cherish the physical sunlight, we also cherish our inner light and celebrate our essence. The summer solstice provides us with energy and serves as a powerful portal for us to infuse light into the beginnings of a new season of life.

SUMMER REFLECTION

1. The first part of this ritual is a journal exercise. Reflect on the aspects of yourself you want to embrace more. Think about how you can bring these parts of yourself forward into the light, and celebrate your unique essence.

2. You can also ask yourself some of the questions from the Solar Plexus Chakra Reflection (p. 75) as a way of checking in on how these themes are operating in your life.

3. Diffuse peppermint oil, and enjoy a ginger and lemon tea as you reflect on your journaling exercise.

INNER ESSENCE CONNECTION

1. Use your reflection notes to make a list of the ways in which you plan to own your power more, connect to your essence, and integrate this into your life.

2. Safely burn the list in a fire or by using a candle. As you watch the list go up into flames, feel your inner essence fueled by the flames to celebrate being more of yourself during this season and thereafter.

FALL

The fall equinox marks a balance between day and night and is the official start of my favorite season. After the equinox, the days slowly get darker until we reach the winter solstice, the darkest day of the year. As fall temperatures cool down, Mother Nature slows down and the natural cycles of decay begin. Leaves turn brown and the landscape starts to shift with inevitable loss. Contrarily, this is also the season of harvest and bounty. Thus, there is a paradox to fall's energy, just as there is a paradox to each of us. We can harvest the energetic fruits of our labor from spring and summer all while seeing certain energies wither, fade, and even die.

Fall is associated with the root chakra and signifies a time to tend to our innermost basic needs: our homes, nourishment, our bodies, and the things that "root" us or ground us after the high energy of summer. Just as in the spring, we'll take steps to bring balance and order back to our lives, clearing aspects of our homes and lives to bring order, balance, and harmony. As spring offers the energy of going outward, its opposing season offers the energy of going inward. With the days slowly getting darker, we may wish to change up our daily routine so we make the most of daylight earlier in the day. We may socialize less outdoors and spend more cozy evenings at home.

This is a season when we can enjoy more chakra-balancing or energy-cleansing baths, meditation, journal reflecting, and yin activities like yoga. We can shift our exercise from the high-energy cardio of summer to more leisurely and earthy activities, such as going on hikes where we can take in the changing landscape of Mother Nature while getting some vitamin D and fresh air.

Prepping our immune systems for the inevitable cold and flu season, which starts around this time, is important. Eating more root vegetables, especially those whose colors resemble the shades of the changing leaves, connects us to the energies of this season and the root chakra. Beets, turnips, potatoes, parsnips, sweet potatoes, onions, and garlic are all packed with a high concentration of anti-oxidants and contain vitamins A, B, and C and iron, which will all give your immune system a much-needed boost. Fall is a time to fall into alignment and balance, to be grounded by taking care of the basics, to enjoy the beauty of the changing landscape and our lives, and to trust this energy process.

✿ FALL EQUINOX RITUAL

CHAKRA:
Root

WHEN:
The day before
and the day of
the fall equinox

TIME:
1 hour per day

The fall equinox symbolizes balance and order, and as we welcome the season of fall, this equinox asks us to be grounded and rooted and to bring balance and order to our lives as we embrace the final few months of the calendar year.

THE DAY BEFORE THE FALL EQUINOX

1. Take some time to journal and reflect on what you might like to release at this time. What can literally fall away with the new season? What is decaying, dying, or outdated? Ask yourself what else you can do to bring balance and order into your life. What would make you feel more grounded and rooted? You can also pull questions from the Root Chakra Reflection (p. 43).

2. Referring to your journal notes, take the time to come up with a to-do list with practical actions you can take that will bring order and balance to your home and your life, taking care of all the essential matters.

ON THE DAY OF THE FALL EQUINOX

1. Go out for a mindful walk in nature, taking the time to really connect to the natural world with your senses: Notice changes in the color of the leaves, feel the crisper air, and smell the scents of the season. By doing all this with mindfulness and intention, you will ground yourself, bringing balance to your root chakra.

2. When you return home, cook some root vegetables. Either roast, steam, sauté, or boil them and make a soup. Get settled in your sacred space, diffuse some frankincense oil, and carry out the Grounding Breath Meditation (p. 169).

WINTER

Winter officially starts with the winter solstice, the darkest day of the year. It's a time when things stop growing or blooming, and there is a conclusion to the cycle of decay that began in the fall. With the darker days can come a sense of bleakness, which is heightened by the stark and stripped-bare landscape. Life can feel unmoving and empty during the winter, both in the natural world and in our own lives, but there is a beauty to the barrenness we see and experience at this time.

Just as animals go into hibernation at this time, winter encourages us to do the same. The colder temperatures and harsher elements entice us to stay indoors, and darker days mean we can feel less like being lively and active and more inclined to rest and relax in a cozy environment.

In the quiet and stillness of winter, with a bare canvas, we can take much-needed time to rest and recuperate, to look deeper inward and sit with both the darkness of the season and the darkness that exists within us. It's a powerful time to understand where and how we may be taking up shadow traits, or our unconscious traits, so we can transmute shadow into light.

As this season is most connected to our third eye and crown chakras, it is a powerful time to embrace divine feminine energy and adopt a more yin approach to life: doing less and being more. It is in this time of stillness and silence that we can tap into our innate wisdom and intuition through meditation, journaling, and visualization, and use our dreams to guide us forward.

While we may concentrate more on our spiritual and emotional work in winter, we should also take care of our physical bodies. It is important for our immune system to get sufficient amounts of vitamin D, so making the most of winter sun and being outdoors, elements permitting, is important to help stave off any winter colds or flu. This can also be very grounding for us, providing energetic balance and connecting us to Earth at a time when we find ourselves more engaged with our upper spiritual chakras.

Hot yoga and restorative yin yoga are wonderful practices during winter. Taking lots of Chakra-Balancing Baths (p. 179) and drinking hot teas with lavender, chamomile, and rose can help you align with the restful energies of this season. Embrace the opportunity to be still, rest, restore, and regenerate yourself during winter, knowing that it serves a powerful purpose in your life. Just as the cycles of nature are operating deep under the surface for the inevitable rebirth in spring, so too does the next season of our lives unfold deep within our consciousness.

☖ WINTER SOLSTICE RITUAL

CHAKRAS:
Third eye
and crown

WHEN:
On the day
of the winter
solstice

TIME:
1.5 hours

The winter solstice is the darkest day of the year and marks the official start of winter. This is a time when the natural world and the cosmos join forces to encourage us to reflect and regenerate. The winter solstice asks us to look inward and connect to and balance the upper chakras, specifically the third eye and the crown.

1. Smudge your sacred space and yourself. Diffuse some sandalwood oil.

2. Complete the Brow Chakra Visualization (p. 127) and Crown Chakra Visualization (p. 147).

3. Make some tea (perhaps fresh mint or lavender), and with some of your brow and crown chakra stones either nearby or in one hand, take note of any observations or experiences you had during the chakra visualizations, specifically with regards to any imbalances or blockages.

4. Write a list of any darkness you would like to release from your life. Perhaps these are shadow elements within you or are about a situation or feelings you have. Let the seasonal darkness reveal any darkness within your life so you can release it into the light.

5. Light a candle and safely burn the list using its flame. As you watch the list burn in the light of the candle, set an intention for the darkness you are releasing to be transmuted into light over the next season.

6. Take a cleansing shower (see the Energy Healing Shower Meditation on p. 177) to continue to release any negativity and darkness.

MOON AS OUR GUIDE

Just as the seasons provide us with a blueprint for our lives, so too does the moon act as our guide. The moon was a guiding force for ancient people, seeing it as a form of timekeeping beyond days (for which they used the sun) and as a way to mark months.

The moon controls the ocean tides with its gravitational force. Tides are highest during the full and new moons. Human beings are made of 60 to 70 percent water, so it follows that the moon's gravitational pull affects us too. For example, full moons are a highly energized time when there are statistically more incidents of mental health issues and crime, showing a relationship between our mental state and the highly energetic peak of the lunar cycle. This does not mean that full moons are bad times, but simply highly energized times. There are also often more births and conceptions during full moons.

Our ancestors did not have the modern-day assistance of our technological advancements; they relied only on nature's cycles, including moon phases. They looked to the moon's cycle to decide when to plant or harvest certain crops and how to work with and navigate the ocean. They understood that eclipses brought great changes, and they knew someone (often a leader) or something would be eclipsed, bringing about an end for a new beginning.

❀ NEW MOON RITUAL

CHAKRAS:
Root, sacral, and
solar plexus

WHEN:
On the day of or
the day after a
new moon

TIME:
45 minutes
to 1 hour

A new moon heralds the start of the new lunar cycle. The meeting of the sun and the moon offers us an opportunity to turn the page and embrace a fresh start. As the skies are dark at a new moon, a blank canvas is created upon which we can set our intentions for the month ahead.

1. Look at the astrological sign in which the new moon is falling and the themes governed by that sign.

2. Journal and reflect on these themes in your life.

3. Draw up a manifesting list, with five to ten items, for the lunar month ahead based on your reflections on these themes. Place this list safely in your sacred space with some of your root and solar plexus stones placed on top of it.

4. Practice the Mindful Manifesting Visualization (p. 167) to visualize your new moon list desires coming to fruition.

❦ FULL MOON RITUAL

CHAKRAS:
Sacral, heart,
and throat

WHEN:
On the evening
before the
full moon

TIME:
45 minutes
to 1 hour

The full moon symbolizes the peak of the lunar cycle and is a highly energized time. There is no better time for matters to draw to a close than under the fullness of the moon. Allow the moonlight to illuminate what you need to pay attention to and perhaps what you need to bring closure or healing to.

1. On the evening before the full moon, gather some of your polished root and sacral chakra stones, place them in a bowl with some salt for a few minutes, and then wash them under running water.

2. Place these crystals in a mason jar with filtered water, and screw the lid on. Leave the jar outside under the moonlight (if you have an outdoor space) or by a moonlit window.

3. Smudge your sacred space and yourself, then diffuse lavender oil. Massage a few drops of the Peace of Mind Blend (p. 40) or lavender oil into your temples and wrists before settling in for a journal reflection exercise.

4. In your journal, write an entry that reflects upon the themes of the full moon. (Look at the astrological sign in which the full moon is falling and the themes governed by that sign in the natural zodiac.) Jot down anything you wish to bring to completion, to celebrate, to clear, and to heal.

5. Go out under the moonlight (if you have an outside space and weather permitting), and read your list aloud.

6. Dispose of your list by safely burning it using the flame of a candle, or you can simply tear it up. Make sure to connect with and feel the energies of what you are releasing.

7. Enjoy a Chakra-Balancing Bath (p. 179) for your root and sacral chakras with the appropriate essential oils and stones.

8. Drink your moon water, infused with the healing and balancing energies of your gems of choice, to complete the ritual.

APPENDIX
MY DAILY WELLNESS RITUAL

MORNING

_____

_____

_____

TIME NEEDED:
_____

MIDDAY

_____

_____

_____

TIME NEEDED:
_____

EVENING

_____

_____

_____

TIME NEEDED:
_____

RESOURCES

SOULSTROLOGY

soulstrology.com

For an easy, practical understanding of astrology with monthly guides and customized rituals for each new and full moon, major astrological event, and season.

THE ALCHEMY STORE

thealchemystore.com

For Reiki-charged chakra candles with custom sound bath meditations, Reiki-charged essential oils, and flower essence aura sprays to use in rituals and meditation.

ALCHEMY ZINE

www.alchemywithambi.com/monthly-zine

Join Ambi's monthly newsletter for tips, tools, and recommendations for your personal wellness journey.

INDEX

ACKNOWLEDGMENTS

To my teacher, Noelle Rose, for all her wisdom, love, and healing. Jamie for helping me get on the right path and keeping me aligned. My brother for keeping my feet on the ground and making me laugh. Mum for your love and keeping me on my toes. Dad for being my protector and guide always. Andrea for taking care of me, my son, and my husband during this writing process. Sal, my best friend for thirty plus years, and all the Deysels, Phillips, and Cheeses for being my "framily." Tanya and Kyle for your unconditional friendship and company, and for carrying the weight of so much of what I do. And Jon for being my soul brother and conscious co-creator.

And last but not least, my husband, Kevin, for being my biggest cheerleader and being so endlessly supportive and patient, and our angel baby boy, Asher, for being the proof that aligning your chakras results in miracles! I am so lucky to love and be loved by you all and to laugh with you all!

To Meg, Debbie, and the entire team at Penguin Random House for all your support and guidance during this writing process and your magical editing skills.

ABOUT THE AUTHOR

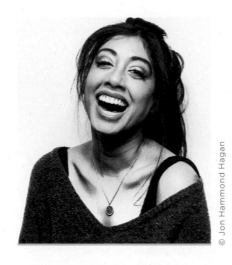

© Jon Hammond Hagan

AMBI KAVANAGH is a Reiki master, astrologer, sound healer, life coach, and host of the podcast *Alchemy with Ambi*. With a unique focus on using astrological cycles and the seasons as a form of coaching, she considers herself a modern-day alchemist (or cosmic change agent) who serves as a catalyst for positive change in people's lives. Ambi went through her own journey of healing and aligning her chakras and saw her path transform both professionally and personally from being a lawyer who lives in London to her life now in America. Ambi lives in Los Angeles with her husband, Kevin, and son, Asher.

WWW.ALCHEMYWITHAMBI.COM
Instagram: @ALCHEMYAMBI